CHRIS GE...

The Cancer
Survivors'
Club

A collection of inspirational
and uplifting survival stories

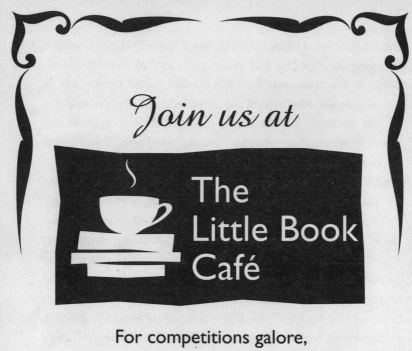

A Oneworld Book

This edition first published by Oneworld Publications, 2015

Copyright © Chris Geiger 2013, 2015

The moral right of Chris Geiger to be identified as the
Author of this work has been asserted by him in accordance
with the Copyright, Designs, and Patents Act 1988

ISBN 978-1-78074-726-2
ISBN 978-1-78074-727-9 (eBook)

Typeset by Tetragon, London
Printed and bound in Great Britain by Clays Ltd, St Ives plc

Oneworld Publications
10 Bloomsbury Street
London WC1B 3SR
England

CONTENTS

Preface to the Revised Edition   vii

Acknowledgements   ix

Foreword by Christopher Streets   xiii

Introduction   xv

Dear Tumour · Chris Geiger   1

In Sickness and in Health · Claire Duffett   9

I'm a Statistic of One · Ali Stunt   18

The Cancer Card · Katie Patterson   23

My Journey · Jason Edgar   39

Cough Please · Chris Geiger   48

Animal Therapy · Kate Beynon   51

Life and Death Inside Me · Jessica Smith   63

A Bright Light · Marilyn Taylor   70

A Father's Perspective · Michael Stephenson   76

Things Happen for a Reason · Andrea Paine   86

Mad Dogs and Englishmen · Chris Geiger   99

Live Life to the Full · Paula Glass   102

If in Doubt, Persevere · Julie King   115

How to Solve a Problem like my Rear · Mark Davies   122

CONTENTS

Never Give Up · Amanda Baird   136

Miracles Do Happen · Helen Gorick   143

Flowers, Cakes and Cotton Buds · Chris Geiger   156

Better You than Me · Abbie Sparks   159

Mother of All Surgeries · David Mason   166

A Mother's Perspective · Gillian Metcalfe   181

How It Was · Barbara Conway   186

Saliva, Chopped Pork and Divorce · Chris Geiger   199

Keep Smiling · Mark Gillett   202

Too Frightened to Ask · Kathleen Giles   206

Getting the Gist · Stewart Hodge   212

A Weighty Problem · Chris Geiger   217

Cancer Is a Word, Not a Sentence · Shelly Ostrouhoff   220

Guinness World Record Newspaper Feature   226

Getting Involved   231

Cancer-related Websites & Blogs   235

Survivors Update   239

PREFACE
TO THE REVISED EDITION

Welcome to the Revised Edition of *The Cancer Survivors Club* book. This astonishing, crazy and sometimes frustrating journey started as nothing more than a self-published project, as a result of my being diagnosed with cancer many years ago. It soon became one of the best-selling cancer survival books. I'd always been convinced that, if I could get this book in the hands of anyone touched by cancer, it would offer them great support, hope and comfort. My only problem was proving that to a publisher. Within just a few months both the response from readers and book sales had exceeded my wildest dreams. Soon I was receiving an almost daily stream of messages – from cancer patients saying how it had encouraged them to continue and even start their treatment again, and also from other survivors sending me their courageous and inspiring stories. I soon started travelling the country, meeting patients, giving talks and appearing on regional radio stations. I was also invited to be the keynote speaker at a large European pharmaceutical conference, to talk about my survival from cancer and how data analysis provided by statistical programmers is a vital and overlooked aspect of the fight against serious diseases.

Now, thanks to the incredible generosity and power of Oneworld, who instantly recognized how beneficial this book could be to anyone touched by cancer, it is now available to a much broader audience than I would ever have been able to reach through self-publishing.

ACKNOWLEDGEMENTS

M y recovery from cancer and the creation of this book are both very similar; I would not have achieved either without help.

Without the medical brilliance of surgeons, doctors and nurses, or the love and support of my parents, Anne and Roger, and my sister Julie, I would not be here now. I will also always be exceptionally grateful to my numerous friends who made me laugh when I wanted to cry and kept me going when I wanted to quit.

I feel equally indebted to the loyal readers of my newspaper columns, who submitted their inspiring survival stories. The task of selecting which stories I included in this first of hopefully many editions was a time-consuming and challenging undertaking. Those who have been selected have won the storyteller's equivalent of Willy Wonka's golden ticket. That's how I think of it, like Willy Wonka inviting people to his chocolate factory; I'm privileged to welcome these people to the cancer survivors club. My job of editing and polishing the stories was made more pleasurable with the knowledge that these poignant personal accounts cannot fail to move and encourage all those who read them.

A monumentally big thanks to Diane Mowlam, Paul Anderson and all the staff at Gravity London for their marketing expertise and designing a brilliant book cover for the first edition; I've no idea how they tolerated my endless barrage of crazy suggestions.

My thanks must also go to Christopher Streets, for taking time out of his busy schedule to write a very nice foreword at such short notice; this means a lot to me.

I owe an extremely special and massive thanks to my terrific and beautiful wife, Catherine. She somehow demonstrated amazing patience, listening to me talk about nothing but this book for months and communicating with the contributors on my behalf. She kept me fed and watered and thankfully discouraged me from calling this book 'Bums, Boobs and Spicy Noodles'. I'd have still been writing this now...

Obviously, I must thank my two fluffy friends Dempsey and Sweetie, who kept me company in the middle of the night and insisted on sitting on any discarded pages that fell under my desk. Sadly, since the first edition was published, we have had to say goodbye to Sweetie, who is sorely missed.

It also goes without saying that I appreciate the opportunity Oneworld Publications has given me, in propelling this book to the next level.

Lastly, thank you to every survivor who submitted their amazing stories of courage. I'm so sorry I was unable to include them all. Thank you to my readers for their incredible support and loyalty. Please keep those tweets and emails coming!

To everyone else reading this book, it's not too late to help. If you enjoy or are inspired by these reassuring and sometimes heart-breaking experiences, please do me a small favour and recommend this book.

FOREWORD

When I was a medical student, oh so many years ago now, I remember one of my lecturers telling us an amazing fact. During an average lifetime, the body's immune system will fight and overpower at least one hundred cancers. These abnormal cells are produced as part of our natural cellular repair cycles, yet they are efficiently controlled without our awareness or recourse to medical help. In this respect, we humans are programmed to and indeed are capable of beating cancer. While this 'mopping-up' of cancer cells occurs continuously and subconsciously, unfortunately, all too often, an individual may experience one cancer too many. It is at this point that the conscious 'survival instinct' needs to kick in and, thus, in my mind, all patients with the diagnosis of cancer are 'survivors'.

From the time that I investigate my patients' symptoms, relay the diagnosis to them and then plan a potentially gruelling treatment regimen, which may involve chemotherapy, radiotherapy and surgery, they are all fighting for survival.

Many will meet this challenge head on, drawing upon both their physical and psychological strengths. I never cease to be impressed by the fortitude and positive attitude of cancer patients towards their diagnosis and treatment. I have a saying that 'You are only as ill as you feel', and many of my patients eventually enjoy telling me about their recovery. Thankfully, most participate in walking, swimming, running and other physical exercise that places them back among their peers. This activity generates a real sense of purpose and a return to normality.

I first met Chris Geiger in the summer of 2010. I was planning a fundraising event to raise levels of fitness in patients diagnosed with oesophago-gastric cancer prior to their embarking upon treatment. His personal story, natural charisma and boundless enthusiasm resulted in that event being taken to a completely new level. Having read his newspaper columns and articles about his other ventures, I believe this book is a natural progression of his wish as a cancer ambassador to get the message out there that 'Yes, you can beat cancer!'

I fully appreciate that cure may not be the end point for all patients with cancer, but this book tells the truly humbling tales of individuals who have beaten their cancer and thus can be considered members of 'The Cancer Survivors Club'. Their stories can now flow to inspire a future generation of patients, friends, family members and carers to tackle the diagnosis with as positive an approach as possible.

Christopher Streets – Consultant Surgeon
The Oesophago-gastric Surgical Unit
Bristol Royal Infirmary

INTRODUCTION

When I was first diagnosed, I spent hours scouring bookshops, desperately hunting for books written by people who had fought and survived cancer. Most of the books I found had been ghost written for film stars. The majority dedicated considerable time to mentioning their celebrity friends or the location of their next film, yet spent little or no time describing their treatment and more importantly how they survived.

Ironically, coincidently or probably luckily for me, the night before I was diagnosed with Non-Hodgkin Lymphoma, I watched a film about Bob Champion, a jump jockey who fought and won his battle with cancer, and then amazingly went on to win the Grand National. The film was based on the book called *Champion's Story*, which he wrote with his friend Jonathan Powell. Little could Bob know that his story would create an idea to inspire me. Watching his film kept me fighting despite my diagnosis and ultimately led me to write a book.

I had to endure two years of cancer treatment. This included a number of operations, radiotherapy, chemotherapy and a bone marrow transplant before I was finally in remission. A mantra I chanted daily during my treatment was: 'If Bob Champion can do it, so can I', along with 'Why me?', 'F**k cancer', and many other unrepeatable things.

I'm convinced having a target, being positive and having the distraction of writing every day got me through my treatment. I wrote a diary daily, creating a light-hearted memoir, recording my thoughts, feelings and treatment; one day I hope it will be published too! I also continued dreaming that, like Bob's, my story would be made into a film.

Within weeks I was back at work again, trying to act as if the previous two years hadn't happened. Any ideas of writing a cancer survival book were purposely forgotten. Not because I didn't care, but every time I relived events, I instantly smelt those disinfected hospital wards, tasted the chemotherapy or pictured the faces of those poor patients who weren't as lucky as me. Each time I recalled these events, I was physically sick, ruining a good shirt and triggering those awful recurring nightmares again! So it's true what they say, time really does heal.

The nightmare of having cancer never left my mind; I constantly worried the disease might return. Friends joked how I must have worn grooves in the roads with my endless trips to the doctor. Just the smallest ache or pain and I'd be convinced I'd relapsed. Each time my doctor listened patiently, no matter how busy he was or how distressed I sounded. Thankfully, over time my paranoia evaporated, yet the whole cancer subject remained at the forefront of my mind.

I now have only one lung that functions properly, plenty of scars and a struggling immune system; but that's a very small price to pay.

I'm sure the chemotherapy also killed my 'lazy' gene or 'sleep' gene, as well as destroying the tumour. I now can't do things by halves, can't sit around doing nothing, can't waste a moment of this life I managed to save.

During the years I've been in remission, I've met and spoken with many newly diagnosed cancer sufferers.

I do my best to explain the things I did to deal both mentally and physically with the various treatments. I soon discovered how invigorated and inspired patients became on learning the side effects they experienced were normal. I also noticed how encouraging and useful patients found it simply to talk with a cancer survivor who understands first-hand how they are feeling. Leaving them beaming with a renewed determination is a great reward for my time.

Back in 2009, I was talking with a patient who said it was 'inspirational' to speak to a 'normal' person. A survivor who'd been given just three months to live and over twenty years later is still enjoying life to the full. 'If you can do it, I can,' they said enthusiastically, while nodding frantically.

It was then I remembered back to the time I wanted to read stories of other 'normal' cancer survivors, for encouragement and guidance for both myself and my family. So began my personal campaign to create awareness and help patients and their families. This book is the result of one of those projects.

Other projects have included writing a newspaper article on World Cancer Day, for which I received a Guinness World Record for 'Most Published Newspaper Article'. I also won the 'Columnist of the Year' award, sponsored by EDF Energy, for numerous light-hearted newspaper columns, publicizing the disease and cancer charities. I was fortunate to write for dozens of local and national newspapers. I've included some of these columns for your amusement along with my Guinness World Record feature. Sadly, I didn't have room for them all; another book idea perhaps?

My hope is that cancer sufferers, and their families and friends, will gain strength and encouragement from the stories within this book. Ultimately, I hope I'll soon be receiving new inspirational stories from readers that I can include in future editions and increase the number of members in my cancer survivors club.

For everyone else reading this, I hope you find it a damn good read and are left feeling positive. Remember, however frustrating life can be at times, nothing is more important than your health.

One last thing: should the final part of my dream come true and my memoir is published and made into a film one day, like Bob Champion's, can I ask that Keira Knightley play my first girlfriend, Emily Blunt my second girlfriend, Cameron Diaz play Day Ward Sister, Jessica Alba the girl bending down under her desk and finally Dawn French play my sister!

DEAR TUMOUR

MEMBERSHIP: # 1

Dear Tumour,
    I feel compelled after all these years to write to you and tell you how I feel.

I guess you know I was a fit twenty-four year old, who had completed the Worthing marathon and went weight training a few times a week. I guess you also know I never smoked and only drank moderately at the weekend. So why did you pick me? Why?

I had a great job writing software, a nice apartment and a flash car (well, twenty years ago a Ford XR3i was a flash car), so why choose me?

For eight months, I continually visited my doctor. He was convinced that I was stressed or asthmatic, despite losing weight, struggling to breathe and knowing the slightest exertion would tire me out for days.

Eventually, after waking up from a general anaesthetic, having just had an operation on my chest to discover what was causing all my problems, I was told they'd found you lurking, wedged between my heart and lungs. The surgeon sat down on my bed, wiggled my toe and said you'd arrived. He said he thought your name was Non-Hodgkin Lymphoma.

Initially, I was actually pleased they'd found you, having felt so unwell for so long.

I wrongly assumed I'd swallow a couple of tablets and you'd disappear. To be honest, until this moment I didn't know who or what you were. So don't flatter yourself by thinking everyone has heard of you.

The surgeon was a little more concerned than I was about finding you. He said you'd kill me within three months and I had a battle on my hands. Well, thankfully, only one of his predictions was right; you did put up a hell of a fight.

I couldn't understand it when the consultant who specializes in removing you told me I'd need to be brave. He explained how I should try to protect my family and friends from my thoughts and the awful treatment I'd need.

He was right; everyone around me appeared shell-shocked and upset. My mum and sister had red blotchy eyes each time they visited me. Mum always struggled to stay composed, yet my dear dad remained his normal strong, happy and supportive self; on the surface anyway. Soon the hospital was to become my second home for nearly two years.

Friends, teachers and ex-girlfriends all poured into my hospital room. I'd not seen some of them for years. They all acted as if I'd already lost the battle and every extra day

I lived was a bonus. I couldn't understand it; instinctively, I knew I was going to kick your arse.

Don't get me wrong – I was frightened at times. The nights were the worst, sitting alone in my room, reading all the leaflets about various treatments I'd need to get you out of my body.

In my mind, I imagined you as a lump of melting snow – black ugly slush that's found at the side of the road. A snowball the size of one and a half grapefruits buried in my chest. My consultant said it looked like I'd swallowed a dinner plate. You were big, I grant you that.

Our first battle together was with radiotherapy. I needed tattoos so you were hit in the identical place each day. Metal moulds also had to be created to protect the parts of my chest you'd not yet discovered. However, you were clever – you were obviously experienced or expecting this. The radiotherapy did little to destroy you; for ten days, you withstood the onslaught admirably. I was left exhausted.

You'd been ingenious by positioning yourself around my lungs and heart where you knew no surgeon would be able to physically remove you. You also knew that by continuing to squeeze my lung it would eventually collapse and fill with fluid. I guess you were also aware my voice would soon disappear, as you continued to crush the nerves that controlled my vocal cords.

Soon the consultant wondered if a mistake had been made with your name. Another biopsy was required to double-check why you weren't tiring and were in fact growing so fast.

At the same time as the biopsy, my lung was removed and emptied of fluid. As I'm sure you know, unfortunately the main nerve that controls my diaphragm was accidentally cut. This operation and other decisions have caused my breathing to be rather laboured ever since. A small price to pay. I shrug them off as nothing more than war wounds from the battles you and I continued to fight.

Eventually, it was agreed by a number of hospitals that your name was Non-Hodgkin Lymphoma; it also transpired you'd been injured by the radiotherapy. In fact, you had to change your cell formation to survive the onslaught. A sign of weakness, I'm sure even you will agree.

Our next battle was with chemotherapy, but not just once. My age and fitness were clearly a massive disadvantage to you.

Admittedly, both the first and second chemotherapy treatments did little to encourage you to leave. These regimes, however, were having an impact on me: hair loss, sickness and fatigue. I continually had to be admitted to hospital for blood transfusions, but the antibiotics helped me fight the infections I contracted.

Another operation was scheduled, as more chemotherapy was needed and my poor veins had all but given up by now. So I had a Hickman line fitted, not the most attractive of accessories admittedly, but it didn't matter. In my imagination, it was like I was re-arming, getting ready for the next battle. This took place with chemotherapy shipped in from America; if you wanted a fight, I was going to give you one. I was even put to sleep for a week, so didn't get to see you suffer.

Oh, what dreams I was having, thinking of you finally being kicked out of my body!

I continued to do my best to protect my family's feelings while fighting you. I let myself down and cried in front of them once, but on the whole did a good job in showing I had everything under control and hoped you were on the retreat.

Your arrival had actually done me a few favours on the girlfriend front. While we spent every minute of every day fighting, I was having the luxury of beautiful nurses supporting and listening to me. Some kindly gave up their weekends or days off to support and help me, others become lifelong friends and most of them were gorgeous too; so I should thank you for that!

With my Hickman line in place, I continued fighting you like a military attack, with every chemical my troops could find; this was biological warfare at its best.

I encouraged several consultants in numerous hospitals to find and give me drugs that hadn't been used before. I was happy to try anything; after all what other option did I have?

I continued getting infections, needing blood transfusions, even needing a second and third Hickman, which meant yet more operations.

You and I continued sparring like heavyweight boxers, both of us putting up a courageous battle. You withstanding the onslaught of every chemotherapy drug I could get my hands on.

Then eventually came my master stroke. In addition to the chemicals that had been pumped into my spine, to stop you claiming squatters rights there one day, I'd finally convinced reluctant oncologists that a bone marrow transplant would finish you off once and for all. This they eventually agreed to, after seeing you were now no longer lurking and had retreated from my bone marrow. But I had to agree to bomb you with yet more chemotherapy first, which I reluctantly did. Don't misunderstand me, I didn't like hurting you but you gave me no choice. I'm lying, the more unwell and sick I felt, the more I knew you'd be suffering too; this I did enjoy.

I then had to endure the agonizing operation called a bone marrow harvest, where surgeons extracted my bone marrow with what looked like a corkscrew, from various places around my body.

Yet more chemotherapy was then thrown at you; this, as you know, was not my idea.

Each time I was close to having the transplant, doctors felt I'd have a better chance of killing you if you were on the back foot, injured and weak, so they ordered more chemical attacks.

Finally, the time had come and I arrived at University College Hospital, in London. This was going to be the location of our final battle. I knew, if you won this, you'd win the war. This was the fight that really counted. I could see from the various scans and tests that you were injured.

It was now or never. However, twenty months of fighting you had taken its toll on me. But with the unbelievable and continuous support of my family I entered the hospital, mentally very strong, physically quite weak.

In other isolation rooms around me, similar people were undergoing their transplant. They too were hoping to eradicate you or your relatives from their bodies. Unfortunately, some of those I met while I was hitting you with the biggest blast of chemotherapy possible didn't make it. This I assume helped you psychologically, massaged your ego; however, it gave me strength. I was determined to leave alive in Dad's car, not dead in a box.

As you know, the chemicals were so strong I picked up more injuries. The same drugs that were inflicting damage on you caused the need to replace my bone marrow, which had inevitably died; the equivalent of friendly fire, I guess.

My hospital room was on the third floor of an old red-brick Victorian building, looking out over an office where people in suits huddled in meetings; I wondered if I'd ever be able to work again. Below my window every morning I watched as a white van arrived, collecting the unfortunate people who had not survived the previous night. The sight of these makeshift coffins being removed wasn't something I should have witnessed, but a sight I purposely watched. I was determined not to end up leaving the hospital this way.

There were times during this fight when I thought you'd got the upper hand, when I thought I'd not see the next day. Times when I wanted my mother with me so I didn't die alone. But eventually, miraculously, you finally surrendered to the onslaught of treatment and moved on.

For you, that's the end of the story, the end of your involvement with me. However, for me, I had a lot of recovering to do, both mentally and physically. Sadly, I can never forget our duel; but I do hope you regretted picking on me.

Over the months that followed, my body slowly recovered, the various scars healed and the distressing nightmares finally ended. I still had moments where I hid under my duvet and cried. In hindsight, perhaps they were tears of joy or relief; who knows?

Our encounter was over twenty years ago now, yet it's always with me and has changed my outlook on life considerably. I'm convinced one of the things the chemotherapy killed is my 'lazy' gene or 'sleep' gene. I now can't do things by halves, can't sit around doing nothing, can't waste a moment of this life I managed to save. You taught me how precious every day is and how fragile we all are.

To your annoyance, I hope, I spend my time creating awareness by writing newspaper columns about you. I talk to people, explaining and showing them how to cope should you decide to bully or pick on them.

I've dedicated a lot of my time to helping various hospitals and cancer charities raise money; money that's used to fight you and your horrible family, regardless of what person in what country you randomly appear to choose.

I don't apologize for the length of this letter or the delay in writing to you. If you had one ounce of humanity or intelligence, you'd recognize it's just a matter of time before you'll be wiped off this planet and extinct forever.

I hope you rot in hell.

Always your number-one enemy!

Chris Geiger

IN SICKNESS AND IN HEALTH

MEMBERSHIP: # 2

I'm thirty-seven years old and have a wonderful supportive husband and two beautiful daughters, Ruby and Lola.

My story started on 5 November, funnily enough fireworks night. I visited my doctor as I'd found a lump under my right arm. I'd seen my doctor twice before about this lump, and each time I'd been told it was nothing to worry about; it was just an enlarged lymph gland. However, on this occasion, my doctor felt I should be referred to hospital, to have a biopsy of the lump taken. This would finally put my mind at rest and hopefully confirm my doctor's previous thoughts. The result of the biopsy would be available in January, just a few days after my daughter Ruby's third birthday.

I wasn't worried about the results and to be honest I gave them little thought. I'd been busy preparing for Ruby's big day, and we were only a couple of weeks away from celebrating Lola's first birthday, too, so both these events kept me occupied.

Richard, my husband, was away, working in Bristol on the day I had my appointment to get my test results. We were living in Salisbury at the time; however, coincidently, my mum was visiting, so she accompanied me and offered to look after the girls.

When we arrived at the hospital, I told Mum to just put the minimum amount in the parking machine. 'We won't be long,' I shouted, as I got the girls out of the car.

I was still feeling fairly relaxed about getting the results; it was just an enlarged lymph gland after all.

Like most doctors' appointments, they were running late.

The girls were well behaved for once, enjoying the novelty of their nan spoiling them. We had to hang around for a long time in the waiting room until I was eventually called. When I was shown into the doctor's small windowless office, the first thing I noticed was another nurse sitting next to him, behind the desk. I sat down opposite them on a well-worn plastic chair.

I was now getting anxious – just seeing them both looking at me had instantly got my heart racing. Soon I remembered I'd met the nurse before, which helped my nerves a bit. After a little polite chat about my girls and how I was feeling, the doctor without warning suddenly said, 'I'm afraid its cancer.'

I felt my face burn with panic and my first thought was for my two girls sitting outside, not the cancer. It actually took a few minutes before I started to worry about myself or the disease. Surely they'd got this wrong or made a mistake? I wondered. I assumed my results must have been mixed up with another patient; other people got cancer, not me.

The next few hours were a complete blur, while I was sent off for some blood tests and a mammogram. Strangely, it was me telling my mum to calm down, not the other way round. Yet inside I was really panicking, but didn't want to upset her by showing it. I never thought I'd be able to handle anything like this, but somehow found an inner strength from somewhere. This thankfully has continued, surprising myself and hopefully impressing those around me.

Richard drove back from Bristol and we went for a drink that evening. It sounds mad, I know, but I just needed to get out of the house for a while.

I felt like I was having some sort of out-of-body experience, or an ultra-realistic nightmare. This was a feeling that continued for many weeks.

The following day, we went back to the hospital together. I hoped Richard would be able to gain the bits of information I'd forgotten. We met with the surgeon who explained everything to Richard and me again. Afterwards, several more appointments were made for blood tests, scans and an ultrasound. Suddenly, my diary was filling up fast, and not with birthday celebrations this time. Overnight, my life had totally changed and felt so unreal.

On 8 February, I had surgery, a lumpectomy. I'd obviously been worried and frightened but recognized it was something I couldn't avoid. I made sure I had a photograph of both Ruby and Lola in hospital with me, so I'd see their little smiling faces when I awoke from the anaesthetic. I knew I had to keep fighting. There was no way this cancer was going to get the better of me and take me from my girls.

Thankfully, the surgery went well and I was discharged the next day. When I arrived home, the house was full of flowers and cards from my family and friends. Their generosity and kindness was the best painkiller imaginable.

I longed to get away for a while, so Richard took us all to the seaside. The four of us played on the beach and ate fish and chips, despite the weather being awful. I loved being able to watch the girls' smiling faces as we enjoyed time together. I did my best to block out any thoughts of my illness or what might lie ahead. I'd started to get angry and annoyed that this disease was interrupting and spoiling all our lives.

But one thing it had achieved was making me appreciate just how lucky I was and how good it felt to be alive.

A few weeks later, I got the results of the surgery, which showed I had an aggressive form of breast cancer. It was a grade three. The results also revealed that two of my lymph nodes were affected. This was frightening and meant I needed chemotherapy.

On 13 March, I headed to the hospital again, this time to start my chemotherapy. The Day Ward was right next to the Labour Ward, where I'd given birth to both Ruby and Lola, so I knew exactly where to go. Just a year before, I'd entered the door to the left, looking forward to leaving with a newborn baby. It was one of the happiest times of my life. Now I was entering the door on the right and would be leaving with chemotherapy flowing round my body; one of the most frightening times of my life.

The nurses were brilliant and talked me through every stage of the procedure. I looked up at the bag of chemotherapy hanging from a drip stand to see it was bright red, which was a shock. It looked like I was having a blood transfusion not cancer-killing drugs. I was given some anti-sickness tablets, which appeared to work really well. After a couple of hours, the bag above me was empty. I'd successfully had my first session of chemotherapy; I had just five more to go.

Initially, I didn't feel too bad, but as the days passed I started to feel unwell. I kept telling myself any suffering was a small price to pay if it stopped this cancer lurking in my body. I'd do anything to make sure I could be with Richard and the girls for the rest of my life; anything!

The week after I'd received my first dose of chemotherapy, I asked Richard while we were watching television if he'd shave off my hair. We opened a bottle of wine, and then, as if it was something we did every day, we took it in turns to shave each other's head. It sounds like one of those drunken antics you'd regret in the morning, but we weren't drunk, nor did we regret it. Shaving my head actually made me feel better, as if I was finally taking control.

A couple of weeks later, my sister-in-law was visiting, so she attended my wig-fitting appointment at the hospital with me. It was actually an appointment full of laughter and happiness. We joked about for ages while trying on lots of different wigs. Finally, after loads of deliberation, I ended up with a wig that we both thought looked like it belonged on a plastic Lego figure. After a few days, I actually chose not to wear it, preferring headscarves. I got some in a variety of colours to match my various outfits; this idea worked better for me. I also went on a fantastic day out called 'Look Good, Feel Good', organized by the hospital. It was a brilliant idea and I had a great day. I was given a big bag of make-up and shown how to apply it properly, which really helped boost my confidence.

Slowly, I really started to feel different. I could think positively and look to the future. I noticed the sun, the flowers and the beautiful blue sky. I was starting to appreciate and take note of everything around me. I thought things like that only ever happened in films.

The chemotherapy was now well and truly flowing round my veins; it was a bonus not having to shave under my arms or legs. The hair straighteners I'd been given at Christmas remained unused. I could also get ready in half the time now, which Richard was pleased about.

Richard and I constantly joked about my situation; having a laugh helped me keep a perspective on things. His support and patience was totally amazing; we were really putting our wedding vows' 'in sickness and in health' to the test.

The chemotherapy sessions were coming to an end and I was waiting for a date for the next part of my treatment: the radiotherapy. I prayed it would be as easy as the chemotherapy, but doubted I'd be so lucky. Soon enough, the radiotherapy treatments started, I was to have it Monday to Friday for the next five long weeks. As my appointments were at the same time every day, I got to know a number of cancer patients, which really helped. It was nice talking with people who were having similar treatment. There was a group of older men who nicknamed themselves 'Gerry and the Prostates'; they even had a little singsong, which lifted everyone's spirits. I don't think Simon Cowell would rush to sign them up though!

It was explained that I had the 'Gene 1' type of breast cancer, otherwise known as Breast Cancer Susceptibility (BRCA-1). Women with BRCA-1 have up to a sixty percent lifetime risk of developing breast cancer and a fifteen to forty percent lifetime risk of developing ovarian cancer. There had never been any cases of breast or ovarian cancer in my family before. I'd assumed it had started with me. Later, I discovered my brother, dad and both his sisters had the gene; they are all now being closely monitored. This knowledge helped me understand the reason why I got cancer. Also, by being able to give my family this information, I knew some good had come out of my situation.

Finding the BRCA-1 gene had other implications, too. After a couple of days, I made the decision to have a double mastectomy and my ovaries removed. It was a big decision having more surgery, but Richard and I agreed it was the right choice. Strangely, we'd spend more time debating if we should buy a new car or clothes for the girls; but this was a no-brainer really. We both felt that, if it reduced the chances of getting cancer again and more importantly if it meant we'd live a longer life with each other, it had to be done.

Unfortunately, the bills still needed paying so Richard was away working a lot of the time. I remember one day while I was with little Ruby, she said, 'Mummy, if you need me just call and I'll be there.' Her kind, loving comment melted my heart instantly and brought tears to my eyes.

Ruby and Lola have a fifty percent chance of inheriting my faulty gene. I obviously pray that they won't, but I know even if I'm not here for them they have a fantastic daddy who'd walk across hot coals to support and guide them.

My surgery, chemotherapy and radiotherapy are all behind me now. It only feels like yesterday all this happened, but it's been five years. There's not a day that goes by when I don't think about 'The Big C' and what I experienced over the past few years. Having had cancer is something I have to live with or, I should say, I am learning to live with. I never thought I'd have found the strength to go through the treatment.

People often say how brave I was, but I don't think of myself as being brave. I just took each day as it came. God forbid you get cancer, I guarantee you will find an inner strength to deal with it; a strength that will help you to fight and win.

I had one friend who sent me a card every couple of weeks letting me know she was thinking of me, which really helped. Don't be afraid to talk about cancer. Sometimes people shy away from the subject and try to brush it under the carpet; for me, talking really did help.

There were a couple of funny incidents that happened along the way. Once, when we were in a café, Ruby decided to broadcast to everyone that 'Mummy has a poorly booby', which was quite amusing, especially after seeing the look on everyone's faces. When Ruby was little, she would walk into the living room wearing my wig, or I'd find her in my bedroom drawing eyebrows on her own face. Moments like these really made me smile and made the treatment tolerable.

I never thought I'd be sitting here now, writing my story and hopefully providing inspiration to everyone who reads it.

If you have cancer, use this book for hope and make it your goal to have your story published.

I still take each day as it comes and I pray I'll be there for my girls on their first day at senior school, their first proper date, their wedding day and all the milestones in their lives. However, if sadly I'm not, I hope they will be very proud of their mummy, and I hope I was an inspiration to them, as I hopefully am to you.

I'M A STATISTIC OF ONE

MEMBERSHIP: # 3

So I'm told I've got cancer and pancreatic cancer at that. My head fills with questions: 'How did this happen?', 'How are my children going to cope?', 'Am I going to die?' and 'OMG, my husband could be widowed.' The fear is insurmountable. Then the numbness comes, the disbelief and the detachment from reality. People are speaking, doctors explaining and nurses reassuring me. Their lips are moving but their words sound warped and incomprehensible. 'How do you cope with this one, Ali?' I kept asking myself.

Thankfully, my body – and mind, for that matter – both have a remarkable tenacity for survival. This probably stems from when we were a species that lived in caves and sabre-toothed tigers pursued us for lunch; our natural instincts kick in and we develop mechanisms for coping. Fight or flight, I think they call it. We instinctively do one or the other, depending on the circumstances. With my experience of pancreatic cancer, I know I have done both.

The night before my operation to remove eighty percent of my pancreas – oh, and my spleen – I was sitting in my room 'listening' to others again. This time, it was the consultant anaesthetist going through the next day's procedure and what his role was. I'll be honest, I was terrified. Not of the anaesthetist, who was lovely, and not of the cancer at this stage. Nope, I was terrified of having a general anaesthetic. I'd never had one before and I wanted this guy standing in front of me to promise I'd wake up after the operation and certainly not before. He was kind and helpful, but looked at me in a bemused manner.

He obviously knew my diagnosis and the statistics for the disease. I was acting strangely, but assume this was my way of handling the enormity of what was to come – a process of breaking down the situation into manageable bite-sized chunks; strange, yes, but it was working for me.

Then there was the chemotherapy. My only so-called knowledge of its side effects was from watching television or film dramas, which in many cases exaggerate the nasty bits for dramatic effect. So I naturally thought the six-month course of treatment would cause me to constantly hug the toilet and instantly go bald. While I wasn't relishing the thought of feeling sick for months, my overriding fear was losing my hair.

Most people may say it's totally illogical, irrational and plain stupid that a woman with cancer is more frightened about losing her hair. But all those media images conjure up a picture of a cancer patient being bald-headed. I most definitely was a cancer patient, but I didn't want to be seen as one. Nor did I want people to pity me. To me, part of coping was being seen and treated as a normal person. Some of you may call it denial, but I just didn't want to join the cancer patient club. I was really lucky and relieved I didn't lose my hair. The combination of drugs I'd been prescribed just made my hair thin out a little, but not fall out totally. Both four-letter words, but a big difference to a woman who loved her hair. I was also fortunate as I didn't suffer from the sickness I wrongly assumed everyone inevitably got.

The treatment itself was tolerable – just. What I didn't like so much was the chemotherapy pump. I needed a Groshong line fitted. It was a small tube tunnelled under my skin into my central venous, via a small incision in my chest. The Groshong line, through which the pump containing the chemotherapy drugs is attached, can be left in place for extended periods of time; I hated that bloody pump. I hated the tubes and the site of them going into my chest. I hated the fact that I had to carry around an unattractive 'bum-bag' to carry the pump in; to my knowledge, Louis Vuitton doesn't make them! Essentially, I was carting around medical paraphernalia twenty-four hours a day, seven days a week. This brought attention to my condition and didn't allow me to forget it either. After some three weeks, my husband had named the pump Eric – probably to wind me up. I just wanted to get rid of the thing; ultimately, I just wanted to go back to being a normal person again.

I did my best to understand and appreciate that these abnormal situations I'd somehow found myself in were the very things that were actually keeping me alive.

During my treatment, it was important that I still felt in control of my life. The reality was that a team of surgeons and oncologists were in control, and ultimately whether I lived or died was up to the cancer inside me. Being able to remain positive was very important for me and played a big part in my survival. My whole family and all my friends obviously helped me believe I was going to survive and this was just one of the obstacles that life sometimes throws at us.

Pancreatic cancer has such a poor prognosis that I had to think – and still do – that I'm a statistic of one and that not all the statistics I read about pancreatic cancer apply to me.

The pancreas is part of our digestive system. It's a large gland about six inches long and shaped like a leaf. It has two important jobs: firstly, to produce the pancreatic digestive juices and, secondly, to produce insulin and other essential hormones. Despite having had most of mine removed, I'm still able to make enough insulin but have to keep a close eye on my blood sugars to make sure I don't develop diabetes.

After my recovery, I decided it was time to step up the levels of awareness for pancreatic cancer, so founded Pancreatic Cancer Action. I'm fortunate to have the support of many leading clinicians and researchers in the pancreatic cancer arena, along with others whose lives have been touched in some way by this type of cancer. Five-year survival rates for pancreatic cancer have not changed in the last forty years; it's my mission to change this by increasing awareness. Pancreatic Cancer Action is developing educational programmes for trainee doctors. We have also created interactive training materials for practising clinicians where they can claim Continuing Professional Development (CPD) credits as part of the revalidation process.

Each of us deals with things in different ways, according to our own personalities, experiences and upbringing. There is no right or wrong way; we each must do what we feel is right or feels comfortable. While I've not been happy to become a member of the cancer patients club, I am obviously very happy to be part of the cancer survivors club. According to a leading charity, there are over two million cancer survivors in the UK alone – a club that is thankfully growing.

I hope that in time pancreatic cancer patients will help swell those numbers, too, and that each one of them purchases a copy of this book.

THE CANCER CARD

MEMBERSHIP: # 4

R eading a story like mine, when I'd just been diagnosed with Acute Lymphoblastic Leukaemia (ALL), would have made such a positive impact on me. I'm now therefore more motivated than ever to spend time writing about my experience, in hope it gives encouragement, comfort and inspiration to thousands of other people.

Leukaemia, like all cancers, is an awful disease, yet normal people just like me are successfully fighting back and surviving. My dream is that, one day, being diagnosed with leukaemia will be as mundane as being told you've got a cold; so this is my story.

I was twenty years old and having the best time I'd ever had. I'd enrolled at college, passed my exams and secured a place at university. It was June and I was looking forward to spending the summer partying with the girls; however, it didn't quite turn out that way.

I began feeling very tired. I'd wake up in the morning and start my college work, but by midday found myself needing to go back to bed and sleep. Over the next three weeks, I also began to get headaches. However, my biggest concern was that I couldn't drink alcohol without being sick – important when you want to have fun! I visited my doctor five times in less than three weeks, each time explaining my different symptoms. These included tiredness, vomiting, shortness of breath, an increased heartbeat and my limbs constantly aching. The doctor, along with everyone else I saw, put my problems down to 'burning the candle at both ends'.

Eventually, the doctor organized for me to have a blood test at hospital but I was naughty and I didn't go, preferring to go shopping; a girl needs her retail therapy! I'd convinced myself there was nothing really wrong with me and I just needed to cut back on my nights out. However, the following Monday, I was forced to see my doctor yet again, only this time Mum insisted on coming with me. She wanted to make sure something was done. Yet again the doctor arranged an appointment for a blood test and I had to promise I'd go this time.

It was now the middle of July. Mum and I headed straight to the hospital that day, where I had the blood test and we then went home. To my surprise at around four o'clock the same afternoon my doctor called. He explained the hospital would be ringing me later that night as they wanted me to be admitted. This obviously shocked me; however, I felt pleased they'd found something wrong at last. Now I just needed fixing. I assumed they'd probably give me a few tablets or a course of antibiotics and I'd be sent on my way.

That night I went to the hospital with Mum and Dad; I can't remember everything that happened now. I do know I was admitted to ward eleven and was told I'd need a blood transfusion. Dad tried to make me laugh, joking about whose blood I was getting. The blood transfusions actually lasted all night. My parents later told me they'd been called into a quiet room. There, a consultant explained to them that my blood tests revealed something was wrong. I knew none of this at the time.

The doctors didn't know exactly what the problem was and further tests were needed before an exact diagnosis could be made. My dad was convinced like me that I was just anaemic.

We both thought I simply needed a few iron tablets, and I'd soon be back to my normal self. Mum, however, had different suspicions, but she kept these to herself at the time. An appointment with a senior consultant was arranged for two days later, when they would explain everything and give me the final diagnosis.

I'd now been in hospital for two nights and I was keen to get home; I hated hospital beds. I soon started feeling better after the blood transfusions, convincing myself I was just anaemic. I assumed I'd be discharged after the 8:00 A.M. meeting with the senior consultant. I set the alarm on my watch for 6:00 A.M. and had a shower and packed up my things. I remember tip-toeing around the ward while everyone slept, doing my best to be quiet while doing my hair and make-up – important even in hospital!

It seemed like a lifetime before the consultant eventually arrived. By now, my parents, my sister Lowri and her fiancé, Simon, had also arrived. The consultant began by explaining that they'd found a problem with my blood. I wasn't really paying much attention, just wondering how long it would be before I could get home. Then I heard the word 'leukaemia'. I remember seeing my sister put her head in her hands and I felt I should be reacting in the same way. I'll be honest, I didn't even know what leukaemia was. The consultant went on to explain that it was cancer of the blood, but it was curable. The only words I heard throughout the whole meeting were leukaemia, cancer and curable. I remember also being told that the people who stayed positive had a better chance of surviving. I lifted my head and looked around the room.

I saw posters on the wall with cancer and leukaemia written on them. In hindsight, I'm surprised I'd not noticed them during my first two days in hospital. Later that day, the doctor explained that, should I need a bone marrow transplant, a donor would be needed. He asked my sister Lowri and my parents if they wanted to be tested. This did start to worry me; I didn't like the sound of it one bit. Not that I had any idea what bone marrow was or how it was transplanted, but it sounded painful.

That night, I stayed in hospital again and for the first time felt truly frightened. It's hard to explain but I think I was in a state of shock. I knew what was happening, but it didn't feel like it was happening to me, if that makes sense? It was as if I was outside my body, looking down on myself. There were times when I'd forget what I had just been told or I'd purposely try to forget. However, the shock would always hit me again later. I spent most of that first night texting Lowri, who always replied reassuring me and making me laugh.

I was told that I'd need some chemotherapy and a nurse explained how it worked. My treatment would begin on Friday, 24 July; at least it wasn't Friday the 13th.

I was feeling really nervous that morning as I walked into the Day Ward. I soon noticed other cancer patients being treated and started shaking with fear and was close to tears. I thought my hair would fall out the second the chemotherapy entered my body, I was so worried. I sat down and looked around the room. There was a guy about my age sitting next to me, and I noticed a girl opposite also about the same age. They were both already attached to intravenous drips. I can't describe how terrified I was; I couldn't even muster up a false smile. My parents and Lowri had all come with me, and their support was invaluable. They listened carefully to everything I was being told and watched as I was given my first dose of chemotherapy. I was in such a panic I didn't actually notice when it had started.

The two other patients, who were already connected to their chemotherapy when I sat down, soon started talking to me. They were so supportive and kept me laughing and joking throughout the whole chemotherapy process. This helped take my mind off what was happening. They were amazing and have now become great friends.

One of the patients was called James. I remember him asking why I had such a lovely suntan.

'Umm... sunbeds actually,' I replied, feeling rather embarrassed.

'Careful... those sunbeds give ya cancer, mind.'

We all fell about laughing, thinking it was the most hilarious joke ever. Before I knew it, my first chemotherapy treatment was over and I couldn't believe I'd been so worried. Much to my delight, my hair didn't fall out immediately either. It actually took a number of weeks before that eventually happened.

I received chemotherapy every week for four weeks. For the first two weeks, I stayed at the hospital. The last couple of weeks I was allowed home during the day, but had to return at night. Going home for the first time felt very strange and I hated having to go back in the evening. I'd constantly begged anyone who'd listen for two weeks to go home, so when they finally said yes I was surprised how strangely frightened I'd become. The hospital was my safety blanket; I felt safe and secure there. The thought of being away from the various doctors and nurses made me rather apprehensive. Contradicting this, I still couldn't wait to get home and snuggle up in my own bed again.

With access to the internet at home, I wanted to do a little research on leukaemia for myself. I found that there were many different types, and treatments varied a lot, depending on the type of leukaemia. There are two main types of Acute Leukaemia: Myeloid and Lymphoblastic. I had Acute Lymphoblastic Leukaemia. There are also three main types of Chronic Leukaemia: Myeloid, Lymphoblastic and Hairy Cell. Chronic Leukaemias are slower growing than Acute. I was soon becoming an expert.

One day while I was at hospital, I was asked by a very happy-looking doctor, 'Have you been told the news?'

I panicked as, even though she was smiling, I was alone and didn't want to hear more bad news.

The doctor said, 'It's amazing news – your sister Lowri is a perfect match for a bone marrow donor.'

I was so excited and rang Lowri straight away, even before I told Mum and Dad. Lowri was overjoyed too and we both cried with each other down the phone.

After my first chemotherapy session, I didn't feel too bad, but the more chemotherapy I had, the worse I began to feel. I felt sick constantly but was soon given some anti-sickness tablets. Actually, by this time I was on a cocktail of tablets, around forty a day. I didn't care how many tablets I took, as long as they were helping to cure me. By this point, my arms were black and blue from the numerous intravenous drips, so it was decided I'd have a Hickman line fitted. This made a huge difference.

After four weeks, I was given a break from the chemotherapy. I was able to stay at home and just returned to the hospital every two or three days for blood tests. I had to take my temperature every four hours and, if it went above 37.5°C, I'd have to return to the hospital immediately. Within a couple of weeks, my body recovered enough and the next stage of my treatment was explained.

I was to have chemotherapy in some form every single day for another four weeks. This really frightened me as for the first month it was just once a week not daily. The consultant explained that for the first two weeks I could stay at home, and then I would probably need to be admitted. This was because I was likely to feel so unwell and because the risk of getting an infection would increase. This was one of the toughest months of my treatment. Every day I had to travel to hospital except for Saturdays. Mum drove us each morning and Lowri and Dad would come and keep me company during their lunch breaks. Most of the day was spent at hospital, but knowing I'd be able to go home made it more tolerable. I had chemotherapy tablets every day of the week and a lumbar puncture every Monday. These gave me terrible headaches. It turns out I should have lain down for a few hours afterwards, rather than rushing home.

On Tuesdays and Fridays, I had chemotherapy intravenously, and I had a break from hospital on Saturdays. On Sundays, I was given intramuscular injections in my leg, which I really hated. It was like a military operation, with everything timed to the hour. Dad and Lowri would take me to hospital on a Sunday and hold my hand while the injections were given. We even talked about things like what McDonald's meal we'd have on the way home, which I know wasn't healthy, nor did I feel like eating, but it helped distract me from the pain a little.

After the first two weeks of treatment, I was asked if I wanted to be admitted to hospital; I replied with a big emphatic 'No'. Driving to the hospital was exhausting and I spent most of the twenty-minute journey with my head in a bowl, but it was still much better than staying in hospital. I found that having to get out of bed, get washed, dressed and out of the house every day really helped me stay active and positive. This I appreciate isn't an option for everyone.

By now, I was constantly feeling nauseous. I had to focus hard for an hour or so, in order to make myself want to eat. My poor mum would cook a meal she thought I'd like, then by the time it was ready I'd start feeling sick again. During this month, my diet pretty much consisted of lots of water and chicken Super Noodles. It was the only food I could eat without it making me feel ill and the only meal I could really taste. Not even a McDonald's would do the trick. It was so hard sometimes to eat when I felt so poorly; I couldn't taste anything for a start. However, I just kept telling myself I needed food and fluid to survive when I was healthy, so I certainly needed it now. My family were so supportive and constantly reminded me to eat, which I eventually managed to do most days.

My hair slowly started to fall out. I remember Mum, Lowri and a friend washing it over the bath. So much of it was falling out, to be honest, I think it was harder for them than me. I'd already accepted this was going to happen so it wasn't too upsetting really.

Towards the end of the four weeks of chemotherapy, I decided to buy a wig. I had two; one was free from the National Health Service (NHS) and the other we bought. I ended up only wearing them once. The day I brought the wigs home I decided I should shave off all my remaining hair. I wasn't devastated; I actually just looked in the mirror and laughed. Looking back, it was an unusual situation to say the least. My friend Natalie was shaving my hair while Dad was hoovering my head. I didn't want to make a mess on the floor. This really makes us all laugh now when we reminisce about my treatment. I didn't feel comfortable wearing the wigs, so I finally decided not to wear them.

The day after I finally finished my second chemotherapy regime, I had yet another appointment at the hospital. Here I was told all about the bone marrow transplant and what was involved. By my having a bone marrow transplant, the doctors were able to give me very high doses of chemotherapy and radiotherapy too. The doctor explained that bone marrow is the spongy stuff inside our bones and it makes our blood cells.

As the high-dose chemotherapy kills off the bone marrow, they need to put the marrow back. This is done like a blood transfusion through an intravenous drip. I had no idea what a transplant was until then, but was shocked when the consultant said it would be done in just three weeks' time. This news scared me but I thought the sooner it's done, the sooner my nightmare would be over. I was to have two days of intense chemotherapy and four days of full-body radiotherapy, twice a day in the morning and evening. My consultant was incredible and explained every last detail to us in the meeting; we were there for what felt like hours. During the meeting, I was told there was a very high chance my ovaries could be destroyed by the chemotherapy and radiotherapy. So a fertility doctor kindly met me and arranged for my eggs to be harvested and frozen. I had injections every day, which Dad quickly learnt how to do at home. Then, after just ten days, I had enough eggs for them to go ahead with the procedure. I'd always thought that perhaps when I was older I'd like to have children, so this was very important to me. Yet, at the time, I was feeling so exhausted I kind of hoped I wouldn't have the option to freeze my eggs – mainly because it meant yet more time in hospital and less time to myself before my transplant. Mum convinced me to go through with it. She was obviously right and thinking of my future. Now I'm so pleased I decided to do it. Compared to everything else I'd been through, it was a small and painless procedure really.

I now had one week before my transplant, so we rented an apartment in Cardiff. My parents, Lowri and her fiancé, Simon, together with my boyfriend at the time, Craig, all went on holiday together. This helped me take my mind off the bone marrow transplant, which I prayed would finally kill the leukaemia once and for all.

The treatment to prepare me for the transplant began. I received two days of intensive chemotherapy followed by four days of full-body radiotherapy. During this week, Lowri was given syringes to inject into her stomach to boost her stem cells, and once again Dad did this job; he was turning into a right little nurse.

On 29 October, Lowri was admitted to hospital to donate her stem cells – I know she wouldn't have charged for them anyway, poor joke! For five hours, she had to lie still on a bed while a machine filtered out my new stem cells from her blood. Thankfully, her cells were strong and her stem cell harvest took just one day to complete. At this time, I was in another hospital nearby, still having the full-body radiotherapy twice daily. Mum and Dad visited us both at alternate times. It must have been so upsetting for them, having to see both their daughters in separate hospitals on the same day.

Saturday, 31 October was the big day. Mum and Dad, Lowri, Simon and Craig were in the room with me. The transplant itself was a huge anti-climax. A line was attached to my Hickman line and it was just like having a blood transfusion. I felt fine while this was happening, just very tired. It was unbelievable to think that this simple intravenous drip meant so much and was actually saving my life.

Mentally, I found the transplant difficult. There wasn't too much pain and, when there was, my self-syringe morphine pump controlled it. Again there were times when I couldn't eat because I felt so sick. My mouth and throat were painful but oral morphine helped. One of the hardest parts for me was being in the isolation room. But the lowest point was when I was told I wasn't allowed visitors until two o'clock each afternoon. I was heartbroken – this really upset me. Eventually, they allowed Mum to come in early every morning to help me wash, dress and keep me company. I'd not been separated since my first day of treatment and I wasn't going to be separated now; I couldn't have coped without my family. They made sure I wore different clothes every day; I even walked around the room to exercise and sat in the chair rather than stay in bed. This really did help me. The rest of my family, who had moved to Cardiff, visited me as well. We all spent hours colouring children's books and generally being silly; even the nurses joined in. I found this really helped pass the time and distracted me from my treatment.

The consultant told me I would be in hospital for at least four to six weeks; however, some patients had been known to leave the isolation room after just two weeks. I decided to make this my target and made a countdown chart. Excluding the seven days of treatment before the transplant, I crossed the days off every morning: 14, 13, 12, 11... when I got to 0, unfortunately, I wasn't well enough to go home. So the doctors allowed me to go back to the apartment for a few hours each day, but I had to return to the hospital every night. Just three days later, I was allowed to stay at the apartment permanently. The chart really helped me, giving me a clear target to visualize my progress. I remember being so excited as I crossed off each day.

Once I was out of isolation, we stayed at the apartment in Cardiff for a further four weeks, to be close to the hospital and medical staff. I wasn't allowed near crowded places because my immune system wasn't strong enough to cope. Everything I touched had to be thoroughly cleaned. My mum to this day still uses anti-bacterial spray at home as she can't get out of the habit; not a bad thing, I guess. Dad became a 'pharmacist' as I needed so much medication at different times of the day.

After four weeks, the six of us returned to our home and I just had one appointment weekly at the local hospital. After the amount of time I'd been away, it was the best feeling in the world being able to go home and see the rest of my family and friends again.

It's strange how people react when they know you have cancer. Some find it really hard to deal with, which at the time really confused me. Some even avoided me and my family, which I didn't understand. However, I constantly had those I really needed beside me and I now understand that different people deal with situations differently. Most people though were truly amazing. My uncle Alan and close family friend Jan worked at the hospital. So they visited me every day, early in the morning on their way to work.

My auntie Julie ignored me when I said I didn't want to go to university any more. She managed to cut through loads of red tape and get my place deferred for a year. Little things like this aren't so little really, they are huge and are very touching.

My girlfriends Lyndsey, Natalie, Sian and Rachel were amazing support also. Some days, I wouldn't want any visitors, but they came round anyway. They knew they'd make me happy once I saw them. They all visited me at hospital and when they couldn't they called or texted me; I was so lucky I had such good friends throughout.

Words cannot describe how much Mum and Dad helped me get through those eighteen months. I honestly feel I'd not be here now if they'd not provided so much help and love. They watched me day in, day out, constantly making sure that I was OK and comfortable. They made sure I was taking the right tablets and ensured our home was spotlessly clean. It's hard to imagine how helpless they must have felt watching their baby girl going through the whole experience. They kept so strong throughout it all; I never felt alone with them by my side.

My grandmother was nearly eighty when I was diagnosed; just a month earlier, she had been given the five-year all clear from breast cancer. At seventy-five, my grandmother kicked cancer's butt. What a true inspiration. It's so helpful to have someone to admire, somebody who knows what you're going through or feeling. For me, this inspiring person was my grandmother; I didn't have the benefit of a book like this at the time.

I was also lucky to have Craig, who seemed to take the reality of my illness away. Craig was an incredible support. We had stopped seeing each other a year earlier, but, when he was told I was ill by Dad, he joined me and helped me every step of the way. With him I could escape for a while and just have some fun. We spent hours and hours watching films, eating food and playing games. I was so lucky to have his support. Some nights he even managed to hide from the hospital staff and stay the night with me; sorry, Dad.

I found sometimes it was hard to talk to the people closest to me because the last thing I wanted to do was upset them. I needed to find someone I felt was strong enough to listen. Even though I was positive most of the time, I still had worries and fears I needed to share with someone else. I confided in Lowri as she was strong enough to hear it. Not only did she save my life, but she was my rock throughout my whole journey.

Whatever form cancer takes, it is a very serious illness. However, it shouldn't be ignored or brushed under the carpet. My point is to try to keep a sense of humour and talk about it if you wish. I remember laughing so hard at times about things that had been said or happened.

Lowri and my girlfriends had such a dark sense of humour. At every opportunity, if we thought we could get something for nothing or a discount, we'd pull what we called the 'cancer card'. This also worked well at home when we wanted dear Dad to make us ice cream or milkshakes. This 'cancer card' would ensure complete sympathy from almost anyone. Lowri was one of the funniest. At all the right times, she'd do something to make me smile or laugh. Even if it was 4:00 A.M. and I couldn't sleep, she'd still manage to put a smile on my face.

In March, I felt that I wanted to repay the doctors and nurses that had been my family for the past few months. I decided to organize a sponsored fancy dress walk. Over three hundred people took part, walking five kilometres along the Mumbles coast in Swansea. It was an amazing day and I got an immense feeling of pride. I was still on medication and had to be careful as my immune system remained low, but I was so happy to walk and reach the finish line first.

I had my twenty-first birthday in April, and my parents held a party at a hotel in Swansea. Companies that Dad dealt with through work donated huge prizes, which were raffled, raising over £1,000. From the walk, birthday party and other events, our final total was almost £15,000. This was donated to the Lymphoma, Leukaemia and Myeloma Fund in Wales.

When I'm asked what is the most important thing people can do to beat cancer, I can easily say it's staying positive and laughing a lot. I'm so grateful for many things throughout my treatment, but the most important aspect was being positive. I don't know exactly how I did it, but my attitude from day one was: 'I'm not going to die, I'm going to get through this.' I really do believe it is this that helped me.

The last two years have been a hard journey, but now I can look ahead. I have regular check-ups at the hospital, which will continue for the next eight or so years. But none of that matters because I'm still here today.

I'm now studying Psychology at Swansea University and left home last year to share a house with my university friends.

I fulfilled a lifelong ambition, too, by spending a long weekend in New York, which Lowri and I promised each other we'd do once I'd fully recovered. I also went on holiday with the girls to Ibiza to relax and enjoy the sunshine; thankfully, the alcohol doesn't make me sick now!!

No more sunbeds for me... 'They give you cancer, mind!!'

MY JOURNEY

MEMBERSHIP: # 5

I was sitting opposite a doctor in a small hospital consulting room surrounded by medical equipment, trying desperately to comprehend the words 'testicular cancer'. These two simple words continually spun around in my head like an annoying tune. To be honest, five years since joining the cancer survivors club, I can still hear those words echoing round the room as if it was yesterday.

The 3rd of April is a date I'll never forget. It's the day I shocked my family and friends when I told them my news. 'Nope, I'm not joking... honestly' was a phrase I repeated a number of times.

Cancer was something other people got, not me. However, I'm now privileged to be able to provide an insight into my journey, how I survived and what it's like to proudly call myself a cancer survivor.

My story began five years ago when doctors told me I had a cancerous tumour, which had probably been growing inside me for several months, prior to its being discovered. In addition to the stress of my being diagnosed with cancer, my wife had recently decided to end our marriage. We were still living in the same house with our young daughter, but in separate rooms. So the atmosphere, as you'd expect, could at best be described as tense.

As I'm sure you can imagine, this wasn't a good time in my life. Not that there's ever a good time to be diagnosed with cancer. Sadly, I was feeling especially isolated and very lonely at the time and struggled more than most. I knew instantly I was facing the biggest challenge of my life; a challenge I had no choice but to accept.

During the weeks that followed the separation from my wife, I'd been experiencing some sharp pains in my left testicle. Initially, I put this down to stress, caused by both the breakdown of my marriage and overwork. My left testicle had always been larger than my right one, which I'm told is normal. When I was younger, my right testicle was undescended, so I'd had a procedure to correct this. Sorry if you're eating while reading this!

While taking a bath one night, I noticed my left testicle felt really hard, like a stone, not soft like the other one. When I examined it further, I got a sharp shooting pain, which made me physically sick. Over the next few weeks, the pain continued to get worse, so reluctantly I went to see my doctor. I was obviously embarrassed at the thought of him seeing and examining my privates; however, in hindsight, it was really nothing to worry about.

After I'd explained my symptoms, he took a look at me. I sensed immediately that he had concerns with what he'd found. He immediately referred me to a consultant urologist; this obviously increased my anxiety further.

According to a leading cancer charity, there are only around 2,300 cases of testicular cancer diagnosed in the UK each year. So many doctors never even see one case, this may have been his first. I obviously didn't know these statistics at the time.

My referral appointment with the consultant urologist was several weeks away and I was worried that the cancer would spread to the rest of my body. I was having so many irrational thoughts, even though an actual diagnosis hadn't even been made yet; instinct maybe? I was stupidly convincing myself I was going to die. A friend at work said my outlook, or, as doctors called it, prognosis, if it was testicular cancer, was actually very good. 'It's one of the most treatable cancers,' he kept saying. I repeatedly reminded him he wasn't a doctor.

While I was waiting for my appointment to see the urologist, the pain continued to increase. Soon anything physical, like just leaning over my desk or sitting on my daughter's bed reading to her, caused immense pain. Eventually, I couldn't handle it any more, so visited the Accident & Emergency Department at my local hospital. After a short and scary wait, I was led into a small cubicle by a young doctor, who was about my age. He examined me and carried out an ultrasound. I could see the screen, which clearly showed a mass in my left testicle; it looked so different to my right one. I was sweating profusely, yet felt cold and my heart was bouncing around my chest, caused by sheer panic I guess. While I was getting dressed, I noticed the doctor talking to one of his colleagues. Their body language suggested there was a problem. Then I overheard one of them saying, 'It's a wake-up call, he must be about our age.' That's when I knew I wasn't being a hypochondriac.

Minutes later, while still in the curtained cubicle, I heard those unforgettable words: 'Testicular cancer.' He said he was ninety-nine percent sure. I asked a number of questions, and his response was very kind and reassuring. I really appreciated his comforting manner and concern. The doctor went on to say it was highly likely the cancerous testicle would need to be removed as soon as possible. He left the room for a few minutes, giving me time to collect my thoughts. As I sat still on the examination couch, it felt like my heart was going to explode, it was beating so fast. I still felt ice cold and in some sort of suspended animation.

On his return, he suggested I have a chest x-ray. I obviously asked why I needed this when the problem was down below. He explained it was important to check the cancer hadn't spread to my lungs. He reassured me it was standard practice for newly diagnosed testicular cancer patients.

Yet again it was excruciating waiting for the results by myself; I felt so alone. I knew even when I did eventually get home there'd be nobody to talk with, hug or tell me I'd be OK; it was very upsetting.

The same helpful doctor gave me the x-ray results in what felt like the longest thirty minutes of my life. Thankfully, my lungs were clear; there was no sign of any secondary tumours. I could have hugged him but didn't want to add a black eye to my list of problems! He explained that my cancer was the most curable type and the prognosis was very good; everything my work colleague had kept saying. Despite what he'd said and seeing the x-ray as evidence, I still continued to worry. I was oddly convincing myself they'd made a mistake and my body was riddled with the disease. Obviously, now I can see it was probably just shock, causing me not to listen or believe what I was being told. These thoughts evoked so much unnecessary stress and worry.

It was hard to believe that little me had cancer; until this moment I'd been a healthy thirty-one year old. Naively, I always thought it was older people who got cancer; I never once dreamt I'd get it. Soon my thoughts turned to how I was going to tell people. I wondered what my parents would think and how my brother would react. I was unsure what my ex-wife would say or how to tell my adorable daughter. My emotions were all over the place and I didn't know what was going to happen next. I felt totally empty and isolated from everyone.

I rang Nic, my best friend, and told him my news. I asked if he could tell both my boss and ex-wife. Nic had also agreed to talk to my parents as I was too upset to tell them myself at the time. When I got off the phone, I broke down and began crying again, for what felt like most of that evening. Nic visited me in hospital later the next day, as I'd now been admitted. My parents also visited, which was a very emotional moment for us all.

After a number of other tests and discussions with various doctors, it was decided they'd operate as soon as possible; until then I could go home. I didn't want to stay in hospital any longer than needed and thankfully there was a shortage of beds anyway. They'd also said that after the operation I'd need some chemotherapy, which was equally terrifying.

Foolishly, I spent the time waiting for my operation by going out every night and getting blind drunk. I thought this would help me forget I was ill. Yet all it really achieved was to worsen both the pain and my now fragile mental state. The result was I'd spend long days in bed just sleeping off my hangover. My parents were amazing though; they kept an eye on me and visited daily. Seeing Mum and Dad was much nicer than just having my phone, laptop and headaches to keep me company. Whenever I was on my own, I'd have really dark worrying thoughts. Not only was the operation worrying me, but I was also getting paranoid the cancer might be spreading.

I'd been allocated a specialist cancer nurse called Julia. She was brilliant; I'd call her for advice and whenever I needed to talk. Within just a few minutes of putting the phone down, I'd start worrying again. I couldn't kick the negative thoughts out of my head.

While surfing the internet one day, I came across a guy called Philly Morris. He was the founder of the Checkemlads. com website. I also discovered a guy called Nick O'Hara Smith from the Testosterone Deficiency Centre. Both Philly and Nick were so kind on receiving my first email. They helped me understand my irrational thoughts and explained how my symptoms were normal. I started to appreciate I wasn't unusual or a freak. I found chatting online to fellow cancer patients who had survived this gave me so much hope and motivation.

My cancer journey continued. I had my left testicle removed and a biopsy was taken from my right side. This was the scariest time of my life. Thankfully, my mum and her friend kept me company and provided great support. I then had a CT scan to check the cancer wasn't spreading, which as the x-ray had already shown it wasn't. Naturally, the surgery scared me enormously, but at the same time the thought of being cancer free gave me enormous strength. After my operation, I experienced a lot of pain in my remaining testicle, so I visited the oncology team again. They arranged an ultrasound to put my mind at rest and more importantly check the pain was nothing sinister.

I soon met with the urologist to discuss the outcome of my operation. While there, I gave a sperm sample to check if any of my sperm were viable to freeze. I needed to do this prior to starting the chemotherapy treatment, as I'd been told one of the side effects was it could possibly cause infertility, although not in all cases. I gave a series of three samples over a period of a few weeks. The results unfortunately showed that I was no longer able to father a child; this for me was a hard blow and difficult to accept. Yet this news was obviously overshadowed by the fact I was still dealing with cancer.

I didn't like the idea of chemotherapy, but was told it was necessary just in case any of the cancerous cells were still lurking after the operation. Once this stage of my treatment was over, I began to feel concerned about my appearance cosmetically, so I had another procedure to have a prosthetic left testicle implanted.

Thankfully, I'm pleased to say I am now cancer free. I continue to have routine check-ups and my last scan showed

I was still clear of cancer. I'm still officially a cancer survivor. From being diagnosed to the end of my treatment took just over three months, yet it felt like three years. These were the toughest days of my life.

Once my treatment was complete, I attended cancer-related counselling, which is something that I really recommend; but I appreciate it's not for everyone.

Strange as it may sound, in hindsight, having cancer was one of the best things to happen to me. Although my journey at times was difficult, I actually never once lost hope and always had the strength to fight and become a survivor. I view my life and the world around me with different eyes now. I'm a proud dad and have met a new partner, Sarah, who I'm determined to have a long happy life with. I feel like I've been given a second chance and the ability to support, advise and most of all help those with cancer. It's my opportunity to do things that really make a difference.

I'm now heavily involved in creating as much cancer awareness as possible. I've appeared on radio stations highlighting the importance of both men and women examining themselves. In addition, I've helped organize various fundraising events, such as a swimathon and a 250-mile cycle tour. I also became a voluntary Livestrong leader and an ambassador for Above & Beyond. I also attend patient support groups, giving talks and supporting patients.

Most of all, surviving cancer has shown me that, with determination, we can survive; I'm living proof. I love my life now and I'll never take it for granted again or be so disbelieving of what people tell me.

I hope reading my story helps. Always stay strong, and

remember there are other people out there willing to listen, help and share their experiences. Never give up, and always keep hope in your heart.

Thank you to everyone for their care, love and support. I owe my life to every one of you.

COUGH PLEASE

MEMBERSHIP: # 1

I apologize in advance if you're reading this while eating your cornflakes; however, I could just be about to save your life.

I was standing naked from the waist down earlier this week, having a conversation with a nurse about Dennis Hopper's recent passing. I must admit I was struggling to act in a relaxed manner, conscious that, if I looked like I was concealing something, she'd be extra observant while examining me; a little like a customs officer studying people's body language at an airport.

I tried to act relaxed as she explained how 'thanks to the Jade Goody effect' people had been visiting their doctor to have every conceivable lump or bump examined. I found it difficult to concentrate on what she was saying, while standing with my wedding tackle on display, willing her to get on with the procedure so I could get my boxer shorts back on.

'I'm hoping Dennis Hopper dying will do for men what Jade did for woman,' she said, clearly not bothered in the slightest that I was 'ready' for her. 'Everyone's as nervous as hell, like the residents in New York after the 9/11 attacks,' she continued.

Now, I normally prefer the lights out and at minimum to be on first-name terms with someone before getting intimate with them. I therefore thought she'd understand why I was being so abrupt and lacking in conversation. Eventually, the nurse, whose name I'd forgotten the moment she'd introduced herself, issued a volley of instructions, like a sergeant major addressing people from the Royal Association for the Deaf.

Before I knew it, I found myself bent over a couch, while she dug around as if looking for gold or unblocking her bathroom sink. My initial worry was she'd lose her wedding ring, until I remembered seeing her putting gloves on earlier. Then, before I had time to admire the view of the various medical books in front of me, she announced, 'Everything appears fine.'

I rapidly got dressed, pleased it was over and now aware how a chicken being stuffed must feel, not to mention relieved it hadn't hurt.

'If only more men got checked out, so many more lives could be saved,' my new best friend told me, as she washed her hands.

I don't normally do stuff like this on my first date I wanted to joke, but knew she wouldn't laugh.

I was happy to listen now I was dressed. 'If you have trouble starting to pee or need a pee more often than normal, come and see me again.'

I gave a weary smile; 'dead' and 'body' sprung to mind.

As I slowly stepped backwards towards the door, doing a good impression of John Wayne, she continued telling me that 'Prostate cancers grow slowly, but if detected early can be treated.'

I grinned and nodded, embarrassed now at the thought of what she'd just been doing to me.

As I picked my coat and car keys up, she enquired, 'Do you examine yourself regularly below?', looking between my legs as if making sure I understood what she was asking. That was it; I turned on my heels and sprinted out of the room.

So I'm urging all you men, once you've finished your cornflakes, go and book yourself an appointment; it might be embarrassing but it may just save your life.

I received many responses to 'Cough Please', my first published newspaper column about cancer. The two below were my favourites:

'Good on you! Good to put this point across to all the men out there. Men are so bad at going to the doctor yet, as Chris' new best friend told him, prostate cancers grow slowly – so getting checked out CAN and WILL save your life. Go on, what are you waiting for…?'

'Poor Mr Geiger… the secret to enduring a prostate examination or any other intimate examination is to act as if it makes no difference to you that your wobbly bits are on display and to act as if you could walk down the high street dressed as you are and not give a damn. It works for me.'

ANIMAL THERAPY

MEMBERSHIP: # 6

My story starts on New Year's Eve. I felt so unwell. I had really bad flu-like symptoms that lasted well into early March; however, I somehow managed to struggle on. The doctors couldn't find anything wrong and thought I was simply stressed. I wish!

Two months later, in May, I'd finally been sent to hospital for what I thought was a routine chest x-ray. The radiographer asked after taking the x-ray if I had time for a CT scan also. This didn't shock me or set any alarm bells ringing; I simply assumed it was standard practice or perhaps he was being ultra-thorough. What did startle me later was the news they'd found a lump the size of a grapefruit buried in my chest; understatement of my life! Naturally, I was traumatized by the news, but the doctor sounded so confident and explained he wanted to investigate further; his positive attitude had an instant calming effect on me. I remember flippantly making a stupid joke about having a tumour, which I later regretted when he said I had cancer, 'The Big C'. The rest of that day was a blur, more x-rays and various other blood tests. I somehow drove myself home in a state of total shock. That evening, I phoned my family and friends to update them with my news. Spending the evening talking about my situation really helped me cope.

The following day, I received a phone call from my doctor, explaining he'd arranged for a biopsy of the lump to be taken that afternoon. This was to be the first of numerous hospital visits. A couple of days after the biopsy had been successfully taken, I was allowed to go home. I'd have to wait as long as six weeks before I got the results. Things were different in the nineties – no targets or urgency, regardless of the disease involved. These were genuinely the longest six weeks I'd experienced. I wish I could have somehow disengaged my brain at night in order to sleep; my imagination was having none of it.

Finally, the day arrived when I met with my consultant to get the biopsy results. By now, I'd become a complete emotional wreck, my mind playing all sorts of games with me. It was explained that I had a 'nice' type of cancer, called Non-Hodgkin Lymphoma. I didn't know that there was such a thing as a 'nice' cancer, nor had I heard of Non-Hodgkin Lymphoma before. My treatment was going to be a combination of both chemotherapy and radiotherapy, which would hopefully destroy the mass in my chest. I'd also have a few operations thrown in for good measure. If none of these worked, I would not be around to see next Christmas; this was such an awful thought. Just thinking about it now gets me all emotional.

So began the war, a battle that I'd have to fight alone, my only weapons being chemotherapy and radiotherapy. I was now very frightened.

I didn't know anyone who'd had cancer; all I'd heard were stories of people who'd died from it. Books like this one weren't available either and the internet was just a distant dream. Not that I'd recommend anyone believes what they read on the internet either.

Soon dozens of Get Well cards arrived, along with bouquets of flowers and endless phone calls from friends and family members, all offering their support. Suddenly, my life had changed and was so different. I noticed through time some people would cross the street if they saw me walking in their direction, as they simply didn't know what to say. I drew strength from all the cards and good wishes. I received well over a hundred and today they are treasured in a photo album, along with various articles and notes about my story.

Treatment started with chemotherapy. I was to begin with eight courses followed by three solid weeks of radiotherapy. Then unfortunately I'd have more chemotherapy just to finish off. The staff at the hospital were brilliant, especially the Macmillan nurses who explained what side effects I might get and how best to cope with the treatment.

The first dose of chemotherapy certainly wasn't what I'd expected. I was fitted with a line into my vein, which was flushed with saline. Then I was given steroids and an anti-nausea drug and then finally the chemotherapy. The steroids made me so hungry that I couldn't wait for the lunch trolley to come around. I had to have the chicken dinner, which wasn't a wise move on my part really; it's strange the things I've remembered. It took around an hour before the deed was done and the chemotherapy was flowing round my body. On the way home, I was still hungry so I stopped at my local newsagent and purchased half a pound of liquorice torpedoes – another bad move. The anti-nausea drugs were effective for about three hours. Let's just say I'm now unable to face hospital chicken dinners or liquorice torpedoes without my stomach turning!

I approached the second dose of chemotherapy quite differently, on an empty stomach. I spent the next nine months looking at life through the bottom of a bucket. There were times when I thought I couldn't handle any more treatment. However, thanks to the incredible support of my family, I somehow soldiered on. Cancer treatments are so different today and anti-sickness drugs are very effective now.

My hair soon fell out, so what I saved in shampoo and haircuts I spent on sunscreen and baseball hats. The benefits were I didn't have to shave my legs, pluck my eyebrows or keep my bikini line under control! However, the worst side effect was the onset of an early menopause. I'd been warned that this was going to happen. Not being an earth mother, it wasn't a great priority in my whole life plan.

Now was a good time to have all the animals I'd always wanted, but never had before. I loved horses so I got one, I loved dogs so I got one, and I loved cats so I got a few. We lived on a farm, so space and grazing wasn't an issue. The day after I got out of hospital, having had the painful bone marrow harvest, I got my horse. Riding her home when I couldn't ride at the time was one of the most foolish, blondest things

I'd ever done. Oh well, I was always told you learn from your mistakes. My animals were my therapy and I shared my blackest thoughts with them. I had to look after them, so I didn't have time to wallow in self-pity. If the day was going particularly badly, I'd tack up Tara, my horse, take my dog, Kizzy, and plod around the bridleways until my dark mood lifted. Tara and Kizzy became the best therapy ever. I'm eternally grateful to both those wonderful animals, who are sadly no longer with me. I'll never forget them.

A friend of mine, Wayne, once told me that we're all like food on a supermarket shelf: we all have a 'sell by date'. When that date arrives, it doesn't matter what we're doing or how fit we are, it's our time.

Knowing my luck, I'll come back as a chicken sandwich! Tragically, Wayne was killed in a car accident thirteen days before he was due to marry my sister. His death plunged us all into total despair; he was only just twenty-nine and fit and healthy. I'd also just turned twenty-nine but was fighting a terminal illness. I couldn't understand why this tragedy and all this unhappiness was happening.

Christmas was a milestone that I knew I wasn't supposed to see. I spent the evening with Keith, my husband, in our local pub, with a nice glass of wine in one hand and a thermometer in the other. My temperature had reached 39°C; I knew I should go back to hospital for intravenous antibiotics, something that was almost a weekly occurrence. My poor immune system had been hit so badly by the chemotherapy that the slightest infection could be my last.

In February of the following year, I was yet again on the operating table. This time, though, I was having cancerous cells removed from my cervix; what a way to spend Valentine's Day! I didn't even get any roses or chocolates from the doctors, just confirmation that I was now indeed infertile and would never have children.

Twelve months on from my original diagnosis and May had arrived again, along with my thirtieth birthday. I always thought of the 'What ifs?' and 'Why me?' on special days, such as birthdays and anniversaries. Currently, cancer affects one in three of us, so the 'Why me?' I understood because I'd now become a logical statistic.

I finished my treatment in the summer and tried to put everything behind me and move on.

My hair had started growing back and I was feeling stronger. I was still prone to getting an infection so had to be careful. My immune system had taken a battering over the last year and I knew it would take a long time to fully recover.

In the Easter of the following year, I started to feel unwell again. Obviously, my worst fears came back to haunt me. Secretly, I feared that the tumour that had been rendered inactive with all the chemotherapy and radiotherapy was starting to wake up again; all the symptoms were there.

My friend Ali thought otherwise and she went and bought a pregnancy testing kit. Two days earlier, Ali had given birth to her third child; I dread to think what the chemist must have thought! Just to humour Ali, I did the pregnancy test. I wasn't laughing for long though when the second blue line appeared. Both my doctor and I were stunned and soon all those tests and hospital visits that were on the decline started all over again. This time, instead of the Oncology Department, it was the Gynaecology Department I was visiting. It was suggested by the top geneticist that the pregnancy should be terminated, mainly because the foetus would be badly deformed; harsh words to hear. Being extremely stubborn and a typical Taurus, I decided I'd have an amino test at seventeen weeks before making a decision. Waiting six weeks for the results of my biopsy for cancer was hell, but the four weeks it took for these tests felt much worse; my stamina was being severely tested again.

Sitting in the consultant's room as I waited for the results with Keith was torture. The consultant had good news as everything was looking normal and I was expecting a baby boy. I would be monitored closely and would require a Caesarean section delivery; not a problem really.

My guardian angels were now taking care of me. Tom, as we now called my bump, was due on 25 December; another hospital Christmas dinner. On 3 December, my nesting instincts took over. I made sure the calves had plenty of straw and gave Tara's stable a complete muck-out. Once in labour, I phoned the midwife who suggested I make my way to the hospital where they would monitor me. Tom was born at 12:40 P.M. on 4 December via the sunroof, a C-section, which all went well. I was back on the ward in time for lunch; naturally, it was chicken again! I was discharged just five days later. I was so not prepared for being a mother; thankfully, Tom thrived.

Time moved on and I wanted to do something for Cancer Research. My mother-in-law was a member of the local committee, so I decided to join, too. I found myself, along with three friends, Wendy, Betty and Helen, and our mascot, Tom (who wasn't allowed to come with us on the walk), walking the new Severn Bridge before it was officially opened to the public. We had a wonderful day, the atmosphere was electric and we raised over £1,000. A week before the walk, I was interviewed by local media, which was great fun. This helped raise the profile and awareness of Cancer Research locally. I then became secretary of the local committee and began to raise more money, along with all our other dedicated committee of volunteers. I now attend many functions for Cancer Research and have had several articles written about me and my miracle son. I continue to help at various fundraising events, from abseiling and sponsored walks to the 'Race for Life'.

I've also been interviewed for television programmes, magazines and newspapers. I've been privileged to meet many famous people and spent a rather pleasant afternoon in Cardiff with the Welsh rugby team.

As time went by, Tom continued to grow fast. He went through the crawling, walking and talking stages and soon it was time for him to start school. He loves life on the farm and it's a wrench for him to leave his cows and calves behind. Luckily, the local school is very rural and Tom spent much of his early days in school watching the farmers and tractors in the surrounding fields. He could only identify his colours by tractor makes. For Tom, red meant Massey Ferguson, blue was Ford, yellow was JCB and green was, of course, John Deere, his favourite colour at the time.

Just as life was getting back to some sort of normality, I began to feel really unwell again. I was experiencing severe nausea, twenty-four-hour sickness and extreme tiredness. I was still taking various medications, such as pain relief, anti-nausea tablets and of course Hormone Replacement

Therapy (HRT). I made an appointment with the Oncology Department and felt very scared attending on my own. Once again, various tests were carried out, including a pregnancy test. I was asked to sit in a corridor while the staff busied themselves to get all the results together. The next thing I knew, I was having an ultrasound and being told I was once again pregnant. Pregnant again, I couldn't be. I was soon to find out my guardian angels had a worse sense of humour than myself, when the consultant came back into the room and said I was having twins. More tests, more hospital visits and more hospital chicken dinners. Once again, I had to have the amino test, this time though it had to be done twice as no one could tell from the ultrasound whether the babies were identical twins in one sac or non-identical in two sacs. Yet again we had another agonizing wait, four weeks this time. Keith and I decided not to say anything to Tom just in case things didn't work out.

Four weeks passed and we were once again sitting in the consultant's waiting room. Good news: all was well with the tests and I was carrying identical twin boys, who we named Jack and Harry. My family stopped me calling one Richard (Tom, Dick and Harry)! All our boys are named after past family members. Tom was told he was getting twin brothers. All through my pregnancy, we referred to the boys as 'the twins'. This pregnancy wasn't without concern; as I was expecting identical twins, the doctors were worried that I could develop twin-to-twin infusion, which means one twin takes all the nutrients, starving the other twin until it dies. Every week, I was scanned as I continued to get bigger and bigger. I got to know so many of the hospital staff. I was on first-name terms with everyone from the porters and cleaners to the nurses and doctors. I have so much respect for the hard work they carry out, for which they get little financial reward.

Once again, I was told I needed to have a Caesarean section and asked if I'd like to choose a date. I chose 14 March, as this was the only date that I didn't have any other birthdays on. Jack was born first, with a reluctant Harry following a minute later. Harry made such an awful noise as they pulled him out. He was not letting go of the umbilical cord, and it had to be prised out of his hand. They were perfect and both a healthy birth weight.

Tom came to see the boys and me in the evening. As he walked into the room beaming, he stopped, looked first at me holding Harry, then at Keith holding Jack, and then promptly asked who the other baby belonged to. We'd wrongly assumed he knew the meaning of the word twins.

Maybe spending more time listening to the teacher and not looking out of the window watching tractors might have prepared him for the biggest shock of his little life. He looked so disappointed, the realization that his life would never be the same again. Up until that moment, Tom and I had done so much together: swimming, walking and horse riding, all the fun things that I feel children need to experience. It was then that Tom decided it would now be Daddy he'd devote his time to.

I had been home for less than three hours with the boys when I was rushed back into hospital with a suspected blood clot on the lung, which obviously could prove fatal. We didn't have time to wait for the ambulance. Once I arrived at Accident & Emergency, I was placed in a curtained cubicle next to a man who was explaining to the doctors that he had an unfortunate rash on his testicles. I wondered if this would be the last conversation I would ever hear. God, I hoped not.

After another five-day stay in hospital and avoiding the chicken dinners, I was given the all clear and allowed home. Keith brought my boys in to see me; however, one of the tests made me radioactive, so I wasn't allowed to go near them for twenty-four hours.

Once home, we all settled into some sort of normality. Tom spent more time out with his dad on the farm, while I looked after Jack and Harry, along with help from our family. The twins, or, as I was calling them, 'the termites', were into everything; sometimes I got there before they broke things, other times I didn't. They, like Tom, also enjoyed the outdoor life, especially looking after and caring for the animals. I'm sure the attraction had more to do with the thought of getting muddy!

Today I suffer a serious lung condition, which is quite limiting as I get extremely short of breath. This is the result of the radiotherapy being targeted directly at my chest area. I'm on medication to control my symptoms, but I'm also trying to keep myself fit and eat a healthy diet. I'm still in remission from cancer and have regular check-ups.

I dedicate a lot of my time to raising money for cancer charities and creating awareness about the disease. I have been made an ambassador for the cause, telling people about my story and lobbying MPs about the way cancer patients are treated.

We are still busy dairy farming, and I oversee the small campsite run in conjunction with the farm. In the summer months, my boys go feral and they have the freedom and experiences that all children should enjoy.

On 18 May, it was my nineteenth year from diagnosis and boy did I celebrate it. Hand on heart, I'd not change anything that's happened to me. I'm not saying that having cancer was the best thing that has happened to me, but it has made me the person I am today. I'm determined, positive, take nothing for granted and know how to prioritize things in life. Having fun, laughing and seeing the funny side in all situations is a priority.

Before, I was very materialistic, only wanting the best things, designer labels, flash cars, regular holidays and a nice tidy house. After the termites have been playing, our house looks like a bomb has hit it. Those things of course are no longer important. The last nineteen years have been a hell of a rollercoaster ride for us all; it's taken me from one episode or crisis to the other. I suppose I could have given up and bailed out at any time, but I'd not be here now to enjoy the most important things in my life, my boys and my loving husband.

MY STORY BY JESSICA SMITH

LIFE AND DEATH INSIDE ME

MEMBERSHIP: # 7

I felt so liberated when I was finally diagnosed with bowel cancer. At last I was going to get the treatment needed to free me from my weak, painful and exhausted body.

My consultant said how pleased she was that she'd persuaded me to have another colonoscopy, but more worryingly went on to say she'd found a cancerous tumour. She looked up from her notes for a response to see someone who felt like they'd just been punched. Yet, by the end of our meeting, I left the consulting room feeling strangely relieved. I think, looking back now, I was obviously in shock. I remember the feeling subsiding to leave a sense of bewilderment and confusion. While going through my treatment, I once asked a Macmillan nurse if I was going to die, the words spilling out while crying. I now recognize it was just a release of built-up emotion. I never really believed I would die; not from cancer anyway. I credit my strong mental attitude as one of the biggest reasons I survived, enabling me to tell my story.

Anyway, to start, I need to go back to before I was even diagnosed. I was first aware I was ill because I ached so much. My limbs continually hurt and I felt breathless from any kind of exertion. I'd been experiencing these various problems for around eighteen months. My family had a history of 'funny guts', as my grandfather called it. He is in his seventies and had bowel cancer, not that there was anything to suggest I did too. I wondered if I had Irritable Bowel Syndrome (IBS). The aches and breathlessness were eventually attributed to severe anaemia.

After a blood test, I was admitted to hospital and received four pints of blood. For a while, my life was almost on hold but the transfusion made me feel fantastic; within just a few hours, I felt recharged and able to enjoy my life again.

A few months later, I met a lovely man who is now my husband and, after a whirlwind romance, fell pregnant. There was then a sudden and distressing death in my family when I was just twelve weeks pregnant, which shocked all of us. During this stage of my pregnancy, I started feeling unwell again. I simply put my pain and tiredness down to the stress of the bereavement and being pregnant.

As time passed, I focused on just how happy my life was going to be, dismissing all the physical problems; I was pregnant after all. My brother and his girlfriend soon learnt they were also going to have a baby, which added to my excitement. I assumed all the unhappy sad times were behind me and hoped my pregnancy was the start of a new and exciting chapter in my life.

After a routine blood test, it was discovered I was anaemic, so I was given iron injections, which is nothing unusual during pregnancy. Yet what was peculiar was I wasn't gaining much weight. However, despite all my worrying and various problems, my beautiful baby boy was born, and we named him Freddie. He had been born prematurely and was therefore very small. He arrived like he always does – quickly and the wrong way round. Even though he was tiny, at 4lb 6oz, he was perfect and required no special care. His mummy did need extra attention though. While I was learning to breast feed, I was also receiving yet more units of blood.

Eventually, we all left hospital and I guess we looked like all new parents in those first mad but amazing sleep-deprived weeks. I couldn't believe that I'd created such a beautiful perfect baby. Freddie was here, he was ours and he was terrific. However, I continued feeling really quite poorly.

Every two weeks or so, I'd have a blood test and would then be admitted to hospital for another blood transfusion. Mum would keep me company and occupy Freddie. This also allowed Wayne to work and earn a much-needed income to allow us to lead a relatively normal life. I'd lie in a hospital bed while a slow trickle of life-renewing blood went into my poorly and rapidly disappearing veins. I was breast feeding Freddie and changing his wet nappies; I was exhausted. I'd never felt so tired in my life!

Soon, other symptoms surfaced in addition to the constant aching and tiredness. Every time I went to the toilet, I got intense pains; they were so severe I'd have to stop. This was obviously very worrying and I tried to push it to the back of my mind. I just wanted to spend time with Freddie at home being the perfect mummy.

Freddie was doing all the things he should for his age, but I felt like I was letting him down. The doctors were still looking into my continued blood loss. I had to endure endless tests, including an endoscopy, scan and a colonoscopy, but they found nothing. I kept being told different things. First it was Coeliac disease, then Crohn's and then it was something else.

We still managed to go away on holiday. We hired a camp-ervan enabling us to take Freddie with us everywhere we went. We'd even decided to run off to Gretna Green and get married. This was going to be our secret until I was admitted to hospital two days before for yet another blood transfusion. I had to tell the doctors I needed to be discharged by Friday as we'd arranged to get married on the Saturday. This kind of killed the romance a bit.

In October, I had another colonoscopy with lots of seda-tion this time, as the first attempt had been so painful I didn't let them have much of a look. On a big screen next to me, I watched as the consultant discovered a strange-looking lump. I was really nervous and kept laughing a lot. I was enjoying the haze of sedation as I pointed and asked, 'Ha ha, what's that?' Then I continued looking as she struggled with pincers to snip off a small piece of what I later found out was a tumour.

It transpired poor Freddie didn't have much room to develop inside me because he'd been forming next to a tumour. I had both life and death growing inside me – an awful thought. Because of this, Freddie took some nutrients but the tumour took most. When I think about it even now, I struggle to understand why this evil disease decided to grow next to my beautiful baby and am amazed how my body coped.

The week after being told I had cancer was one of the hardest of my life, waiting to hear if it had spread or not. Because of this, frustratingly, I'd not been able to start any treatment and I still felt so ill and constantly tired. It was equally disturbing having to see my family doing their best to hide their emotions. I knew what some people might have thought; I was only twenty-seven and had a six-month-old baby boy.

I was finally diagnosed with secondary bowel cancer, which would need surgery and chemotherapy.

I was so pleased and happy they had finally found the cause of my problems and could begin treating me.

I felt at my worst when I went into hospital for the operation to have the lump removed. The 'Nil by Mouth' sign posted above my bed reminding staff I wasn't to eat anything didn't help. I'd also had to take some laxatives the night before to make sure my bowels were empty. I was at the lowest weight I'd been since I was a child. My red blood count was now just six, half of what it should have been. This meant I needed more blood before they would operate on me. I was feeling so worried and depressed and wondered if I'd even survive the operation. The excitement of them finding the cancer had rapidly eroded.

When I eventually woke from the surgery, I was violently sick. It was a horrible feeling but thankfully a Macmillan nurse had organized a private side room enabling me to be with Freddie. When I touched my side where the pain had always been, I felt nothing; it was such a big relief. Instantly, I realized the lump had been cut out. I knew whatever came next didn't matter; I was going to do my best to survive.

As soon as I started to recover from the operation, I began a course of chemotherapy. Mum again kept me company every day and looked after my gorgeous boy while I received my treatment. It sounds a cliché I know, but she really was my rock. As a mum myself now, I fully appreciate how she must have felt.

I don't want to write too much about the chemotherapy, but looking back Mum always managed to make me laugh, which was so important. She regularly made the three of us a picnic and helped Freddie to learn to walk while on the hospital ward. I tried to pretend we were like any normal young family, even if my chemotherapy pump went off every few minutes.

It's very likely that the surgery and treatment I received for cancer was the cause of my intolerance to some foods. The surgery involved removing my ascending colon and rejoining my intestines. I also believe my digestive system is more sensitive now due to the chemotherapy; but this is a small price to pay. Most people at some time in their life suffer from similar complaints to these anyway. The biggest and most unique side effect is I now have less time to get to the toilet, less warning that I need to go. I'm trying a gluten-free diet, which appears to help a little, but I'm still learning about what my body prefers even now.

It's these things that remind me I've fought cancer, but I am alive and enjoying life, which is the most important thing. I have some impressive-looking scars too; my favourite is my Caesarean scar but the one across my belly button is the one that saved my life. Strange as it may sound, I love it.

My family and friends provided such amazing support

while I was unwell. One friend gave me a wonderful gift of a twice-weekly shiatsu massage. This gave me strength and showed her love, which helped beyond words. I don't regret the experience of having cancer, however strange that sounds. It's funny to think having cancer was actually good for me. I'm pleased to say that no true friend shied away; they shared all my dark times and celebrated the great times with me as well.

Wayne and I don't talk about my experience with cancer much; it's hard for him to comprehend.

I'm not sure he really even understands it all now; I know I don't.

What else is there to write about having cancer at twenty-seven? Don't give up; it sounds so corny but it's true.

If I had given up, I wouldn't have my other beautiful son, Rowan, who is three years old now. My oncologist told me that it was highly unlikely I would remain fertile after all the chemotherapy, but another miracle occurred when my fantastic crazy Rowan arrived. It was incredible to experience a healthy pregnancy, without all the fatigue, blood transfusions and worry. I can now be the sort of mum I always wanted to be. My children are everything and I'm just a woman who is foremost a mother and also now a member of the cancer survivors club.

Having cancer has changed me for the better. I never put up with rubbish from people or waste time doing jobs I hate doing. We still have the stresses and strains of everyday life, but I never forget I'm lucky to have been given another chance. When you've been to the darkest place, there is nowhere else to go but up. Up, up, up and away with the rest of my wonderful life for however long it lasts.

A BRIGHT LIGHT

MEMBERSHIP: # 8

I'm sixty-five years old and my main hobby is gardening, but never in a million years did I think this would save my life.

One day, I thought I'd prune some of the tall trees in our garden. I climbed the ladder and reached the top of the tree with my sixteen-foot pruner. Once I'd finished the job, I threw the pruner on top of the growing pile of branches I'd cut off. At that moment, something in the back of my neck hurt and didn't feel quite right.

A week went by and the pain in my neck got worse, so I decided I should go to the doctor. They said I'd probably just pulled a muscle and gave me some painkillers. These didn't work and my neck continued to hurt, so the following week I went back again. This time I was given yet more painkillers, but stronger ones; again these didn't work either. Four weeks later and the pain just kept getting worse. Then one night I went to bed and woke up to find that I had lost most of the use of my right arm. My initial thought was I'd had a stroke, which was terrifying. So back to the doctor I went again; calmly I showed him that my arm had stopped working. To my amazement, I was just packed off home with even more painkillers. A week later, I went back yet again and this time they still appeared to ignore what I was saying. It was becoming very frustrating, not to mention painful. It was now eight weeks since I'd started getting the pain while gardening and it continued to get worse. At times it was so severe it prevented me from sleeping normally.

During this time, there wasn't one doctor who suggested I should have a scan; I'd now been seen by all five doctors at my local surgery, too!

Each week I went to see them and each week they gave me different types of painkillers, which provided no relief from the pain. I was at desperation's door, so in one last-ditch attempt went back to the doctor. This time, I really did have a good old moan, I was so frustrated and angry.

At last, this doctor made an appointment for me to see a physiotherapist, to see if they could help with the mobility of my now useless right arm. The physiotherapist started various exercises, but the pain they caused was so intense it felt like my whole body was being kicked.

Eventually, the physiotherapist stopped the exercises, as they were actually making me feel ill. She thought I should see a doctor at the hospital. By the time I arrived, I was doubled up in pain. I begged for the doctor to do something for me and quickly. She arranged for me to have a scan. At long last, after nine weeks, somebody was actually listening to me. Just three days later, I was having a scan of my back and neck.

The following day, while I was waiting for another appointment with the physiotherapist, which I was obviously dreading, my doctor called asking if I could pop down and see him. This really started to panic me. It was then I was given the news that I had a tumour on my spine. Words can't describe how absolutely devastated I felt. Immediately, the doctor made an appointment at the main hospital. I was told I should collect the MRI scan results from another hospital en route.

My husband and daughter arrived at the hospital within an hour with the scan results and I was immediately admitted. After months of moaning that nothing was happening, suddenly people were listening and things were moving quickly.

The next morning, I was to have a life-or-death operation – literally. When I came round from the operation, I was connected to a life-support machine. Thankfully, from there on, I progressed and got loads better each day. While I was recovering from the operation in the hospital, doctors told me they'd removed a large tumour from the top of my spine. This was why I'd been experiencing such terrible pain in my neck and back. Thankfully, now the pain has totally gone. I was told I was lucky to be alive. The surgeon said, if the tumour had not been found and dealt with, I'd have soon lost the use of all my limbs, not to mention my life. I was told I had an extremely rare type of cancer and it was even rarer for the spine to be the primary site for cancer. This news was such a massive shock to both me and all my family.

Each day, I kept thinking to myself, 'I'm sure I didn't hear this right' or perhaps I'd been having some kind of bad dream. While I was in hospital I never once thought, 'Why me?' My focus and concentration was purely on getting better and surviving. The doctor once asked if I would like to see the hospital chaplain, which I agreed to. Not that I ever thought I might die, but I knew my Christian faith would help me through my treatment. The chaplain and I went into a room together and she asked if I wanted to pray. As we were saying a prayer, I could hear the chaplain speaking, but lost track of her being there.

As I clasped my hands in prayer, I saw Jesus' hands praying in the same way as me. In his hands he was holding the brightest light I'd ever seen. Next to me in my prayers my husband and daughter were sitting in a line. Jesus passed the light into my hands and then I passed the light into my husband's hands. He in turn passed it on to my daughter. This was truly a wonderful feeling and, although the chaplain was still speaking, I'm embarrassed to say I didn't really hear much of what she said. She asked me if I was all right and I explained I'd seen the most wonderful sight. Afterwards, she told me that she felt I'd received a truly wonderful sign and the light would always be with all of us, wherever we all go. From that day on, my life has continued to get better.

Near the end of my stay in hospital, six of the doctors came to see me. I knew they had come to talk to me about the cancer. One of the doctors said the cancer treatment would start once I'd been discharged. This again was a bit frightening, but I was determined I'd deal with whatever treatment I had and ultimately survive.

I was measured up for a collar to support my spine and neck; I had to wear it for about nine weeks following my discharge. I even had to wear the collar in bed, which prevented me from lying flat on my back. This was because, when the surgeon operated to remove the tumour, my spine had to be rebuilt with a titanium mesh and cement to replace the fifth and sixth vertebrae. This was due to the bone being completely destroyed by the cancer.

I soon received a course of radiotherapy, which consisted of five sessions a week.

From time to time, I needed the odd x-ray just to ensure that everything was all right.

In all the time that I had the cancer, I never once thought that I would die. I believed I'd get better because I had everything to live for: a wonderful husband, daughter, son-in-law and grandson. They were my reason to live, fight and beat the disease.

I've now fully recovered and I owe my thanks to all the doctors and nurses who have helped me along my cancer journey; without them I would not be here. I must say to everyone, if you think that you might have any type of cancer, please get it checked. There was nobody more frightened than me and I'm so grateful to the people that saved my life.

I'm right handed but unfortunately due to the tumour I lost the use of part of my right arm. Thankfully, I can use my left arm and hand to move my right arm where it needs to be, and this works just fine. I have now had the results from my latest tests, which say there is still no sign of any cancer. This truly is a wonderful feeling.

Unfortunately, my husband was diagnosed with prostate cancer in July. This has been a really stressful road we have both been down but now everything is drawing to a close. Thankfully, my husband has also recently been given the all clear from his cancer.

Our thanks go to our family for their love and devotion shown to us.

A FATHER'S PERSPECTIVE

MEMBERSHIP: # 9

M y daughter Clare was having a difficult time during the early stages of her long-awaited pregnancy. She detected all was not well but her doctors didn't appear overly worried. They simply put her concerns down to being an excessively anxious new mum-to-be.

In June, my wife and I visited her at home, just as doctors had finally agreed to admit Clare to hospital for some tests. They wanted to explore why she felt so unwell. Clare asked her mum, Yvonne, to accompany her.

After her appointment, Clare then stayed with us for the weekend. However, she soon received a phone call from the hospital asking if she could pop back in on the Sunday. They explained they wanted to carry out some more tests. Clare readily agreed as she was feeling so unwell. She actually asked if they could see her a day earlier, on the Saturday, and thankfully they agreed.

On Saturday, after a few more tests, the doctors discovered Clare had an ovarian cyst. She was immediately admitted and the doctors proposed to remove it during surgery the following Monday.

When Yvonne and I visited Clare later on Monday after her surgery, she told us the dreadful news that surgeons had actually found some type of cancer. This had been found in her bowel and samples had been sent off for testing. To learn your child has cancer is quite simply the most devastating thing to experience. What do you say when you're asked, 'Why me, Dad?'

During the following week, as Clare recovered from surgery, we all waited for the test results of her biopsy. Yvonne and I visited every day, staying at a small hotel close to the hospital. Kris, Clare's husband, was staying with his parents. We didn't want to intrude by staying at Clare and Kris' house.

The next Monday, Clare was transferred to a cancer centre at a different hospital. We arrived in the evening to find her looking very poorly and breathing with the aid of oxygen. Again we stayed nearby and visited her the following day. Sadly, during Tuesday night, she lost her baby. It was thought the surgery may have been too much for her body to handle.

On the Wednesday afternoon, a doctor had arranged to see Clare. He'd seen her on Tuesday night after we'd all gone, but Clare wanted us to be there when he examined and talked to her again. During his examination, we noticed he looked very concerned. Within just minutes, he arranged for a chest x-ray and swiftly organized for her to be moved into the Intensive Care Unit (ICU). We had been told that this doctor, who specialized in cancer, spoke his mind and was very direct in his approach. But we really weren't expecting him to tell us that Clare was desperately ill and had failing kidneys. We also weren't expecting him to tell us we should prepare ourselves for the worst: Clare could actually die. I can't begin to explain how awful it felt to be told she might not make it. I was standing in a busy hospital corridor outside Clare's ward at the time, with people rushing around, when we were given this dreadful news. I am not ashamed or embarrassed to admit I broke down and cried.

We soon found ourselves following an ambulance to the other hospital and then sat in the family waiting room, while nurses took Clare into the ICU. By now it was gone 11:00 P.M. During that long dreadful night of tears, we were visited by the duty doctor who said he was going to try to kick-start her kidneys with injections of diuretics. However, in his words: 'I don't think we'll succeed.'

As Thursday morning dawned, Clare was thankfully still with us. She was certainly putting up a good fight, bless her. The nurses and doctors on the ICU were wonderful. It's so hard to describe how grateful I was – no tin of chocolates or words of thanks could begin to express just how thankful I was. Again, we had to find somewhere to stay the night, so found a room in a local bed & breakfast. The nursing staff assured us they would call the minute they thought we should come back to the hospital to be with Clare; for the moment she was stable.

We were so exhausted we soon managed to drop off to sleep. It was a wonderful feeling when we woke to realize the phone hadn't rung during the night. However, when we arrived at the hospital on the Friday morning, we found she'd been put on a life-support machine as well as being given drugs to keep her sedated.

Her kidneys were still failing. We sat with her all day, doing shifts and simply holding her hand, knowing she might be about to die. During one of my breaks, I met a man from Scotland next to the coffee machine. His son was in a coma after being involved in a car accident. He asked for our names and said he'd pray for us in the chapel. He explained he prayed every day for his son. In those darkest of moments, I really felt lifted by this kind man's sentiments.

At about 6:00 P.M., I looked up from Clare's bed to see the doctor coming into the room, with another man behind him. He introduced himself as the haematology consultant and said he wanted to talk to Clare. He asked her some basic questions: her age, where she lived, etc. Clare responded so quickly we were all quite surprised. The drugs had clearly worn off by now. Both doctors explained they wanted to talk to us all, so we quickly gathered in a small meeting room next door. They said the results of Clare's biopsy had shown she had a rare type of Non-Hodgkin Lymphoma. Because it was rare, it had taken longer than normal to be identified. They said it was treatable with chemotherapy, but imperative they started that evening. The bad news was her chances of survival were very slim. Now we'd gone from no chance to slim chance; this gave us hope! By the time we got back to see Clare again, they'd already started reconnecting the life-support machine, which had been removed when all seemed lost. Yvonne and I went back to the bed & breakfast that night, clutching at this small window of hope and relieved Clare was still fighting.

When we saw her the next morning, it seemed as if the Scottish man's prayers had been answered. Clare's kidneys had suddenly started working again. I never thought I'd get so excited at the sight of a catheter bag full of urine! Clare had even asked to see her sister Erika and her brother-in-law Jeremy. They too were obviously excited and drove up later that day to see her. This gave her a tremendous boost and again we returned to our bed & breakfast that evening with slightly more hope.

The next morning when we arrived at ICU, we were met by an animated Diane, Kris' mum.

She said we'd not believe our eyes when we saw Clare. Worried, we rushed in to see her sitting up in bed, putting milk and sugar on cornflakes and sipping a glass of orange juice.

Clare appeared full of energy; it was absolutely remarkable. She was still fighting, though, and the slim chance looked like it was getting bigger. Friends of Clare also visited during that day, which again she appreciated. This was quickly becoming the best Father's Day I could have ever dreamt of.

On Monday morning, we were told that Clare would be having an MRI scan at around 1:00 P.M. But first she needed to have an uncomfortable lumbar puncture as samples of her spinal fluid were needed. After the scan, she was to be taken straight up to the Haematology Department. This was amazing news that she no longer needed to be in ICU.

During Tuesday morning, we were with Clare as the nurse gave her the second dose of chemotherapy. Over the next couple of days, she started to drink fluids again by mouth and her appetite slowly returned. I even managed to tempt her with a prawn salad sandwich. But only after I had cut off the crusts and cut the bread into small triangles. It was so brilliant to see her wolfing them down.

By Saturday, she managed to get out of bed and sit in the bedside chair for a while. On Sunday, she also managed to eat a roast lunch and had more friends to visit. During Clare's stay, I was surprised by the number of different nurses who kept popping in to visit her. These were the nurses who had looked after her from the maternity section, ICU and Haematology Department. They'd all come to keep an eye on her progress and regularly give her pep talks, which was so kind. Clare continued to improve rapidly now and no longer needed oxygen or intravenous lines. She also started to walk by taking a few steps to the bathroom.

On Saturday, 2 July, she was allowed home during the day, but had to return to the hospital at night. When we next visited Clare, it was such a wonderful sight to see her dressed, standing without crutches waiting at the front door for us. From no chance to slim chance, she now had every chance of beating this cancer.

On Wednesday, 6 July, she was finally discharged and we helped her move back home. I was so excited how quickly she was regaining her mobility.

A few days later, we all went out for a celebratory meal and had quite a normal evening under the circumstances.

Clare continued to get stronger over the next week or so, but worryingly around the middle of July she developed some really bad headaches. Initially, she put them down to migraines, which she had suffered from in the past. But within two or three days she was back in hospital, being checked over. The doctor's first thought was the migraine had been brought on by stress. They organized a CT scan, which unfortunately showed the lymphoma had moved up from her spinal area to around her brain. When Kris rang with this news around teatime on Thursday, I felt absolutely gutted. One minute we're told we're going to lose Clare, and then she is OK; next, we hear the cancer has spread. I told Kris we'd drive up immediately. Thankfully, we managed to get a room in the same bed & breakfast and we arrived just after 9:00 P.M.; but it was too late to visit Clare.

When we saw her the next morning, her headaches had eased, with the help of some drugs. She kept asking if it was getting dark as she was having trouble seeing clearly. The specialist arranged for a neurosurgeon to examine her, who in turn arranged for an MRI scan to be done. Later that day, the duty doctor explained that, if the scan indicated the need, they would start Clare on some new chemotherapy that evening. He said they had pre-empted the scan results and ordered the chemotherapy from the pharmacy already, just in case.

During the night, Clare had indeed started the first of an intensive course of chemotherapy, and the rest was to follow over the next two days. By Saturday afternoon, she was feeling brighter but her sight had virtually gone. I explained to Clare that we would go home that night and come back

Sunday. Just as we were about to leave, she needed to use the toilet and Kris had to guide her towards it. I was so pleased she was unable to see my face as I watched her being led to the cubicle; it was utterly heart-breaking. After nearly dying from kidney failure, and the trauma of chemotherapy, my dear baby girl was now practically blind. We had no idea if her loss of sight was permanent or not.

There was not much to say as Yvonne and I drove back home. We rang on the Sunday morning and Clare did sound much brighter and slightly happier. I suggested she rest as much as she could as she didn't have any visitors coming that day.

As the bed & breakfast was fully booked, we saw her on the Monday, not Sunday. Over the next couple of days, she said she had started to see strange shapes. As we walked across the car park on Thursday morning and looked up to her fifth-floor room, I couldn't believe it when I saw Clare waving at us; this instantly started me off crying again. When we arrived in her room we found her dressed and sat up in her armchair. She was also free of all lines and drips. What a 'remarkable girl' she is, I kept telling her.

We had to go home on Friday to tend to Yvonne's elderly mother, but later that evening Clare rang to tell us that she would be allowed home during the day on Saturday. The only downside was she would still have to spend the night in hospital. By now her vision was almost back to normal; thank God.

On 5 August, her birthday, Clare was again allowed home during the day but the hospital still wanted to keep an eye on her during the night. Their house was crammed with both sets of family, which I could tell was getting a bit too much for her as she'd started to look really tired.

On 9 August, we visited her and took her for a little walk in the nearby park, making the most of the warm sunshine. Clare was still feeling fragile as the chemotherapy did its job. This was expected; however, the doctors were really pleased with her progress.

A day or so later, we had a call from Clare saying she'd got the results of her CT scan early. It appeared that her body, including the brain area, was totally free of any cancer. Good news indeed, but I was not about to break open the champagne just yet, as I was getting used to having a setback after each piece of good news.

Throughout August and September, Clare continued going in and out of the hospital for various tests and treatments. During November, she had her last course of chemotherapy.

By January of the next year, she was back at home and had to visit the Oncology Centre as an out-patient, for a course of radiotherapy. She was to have this on the base of her head to eradicate any last traces there might be of the disease.

Over the next few months, Clare made great strides back to full health again. Now she just has regular blood tests and check-ups as a precautionary measure, as I know all members of the cancer survivors club do.

About a year later, both Clare and Kris had fully recovered mentally and physically from the experience. Thankfully, we finally have our daughter back and Kris has his wife.

In August 2012, Clare reached the six-year milestone since the end of her treatment. She is fit and well and the dark days are a fading memory. This horrible encounter with cancer has really changed our lives. Clare and Kris work hard to raise awareness for various local cancer charities near their home in Bristol. They even did a sponsored bike ride, which raised more desperately needed funds for charity.

No longer do any of us take life for granted or waste a minute of our days; we appreciate just how precious life is.

THINGS HAPPEN FOR A REASON

MEMBERSHIP: # 10

There it was, the tiniest spot of blood. It was no bigger than a pinhead. At the time, I thought it could be just about anything, so ignored it.

A few more months went by and I'd practically forgotten about my little red spot until it appeared again. This time, it was obvious it was a spot of blood. However, it was now bigger and far more visible than a few months earlier.

I'd started running almost a year to that day. I began as I had a high-pressured job working practically every hour given. Stress as we know can do all sorts of nasty things to your body. Not only did I want to reduce my anxiety levels, but I also wanted to lose some pounds. Somehow, my weight had crept up to over twenty pounds more than my ideal weight. It took me a long time to admit I was a runner. I was a swimmer, but a swimmer that didn't have enough hours in her day to practise the sport. Running was easy: just throw on a pair of shoes and head out the door. It's a beneficial low-maintenance sport. Boy, I'm starting to sound like an athlete or some super-fit woman – I'm not!

A year into practising my newfound sport, I was back to my ideal weight; I was now feeling stronger and on top of the world. I'd even run a half-marathon; yes, I'd managed 13.1 miles or 21.1 kilometres. Then I saw that spot of blood again. It just happened that I was reading a lot of books and magazines on running at the time. I recalled reading about women who were clocking up a lot of miles during their weekly training. Some were experiencing irritated breast nipples, which sometimes bled.

This was caused by the friction of their bra constantly rubbing. I simply assumed the rubbing had caused the spot of blood. After all, I was in the best physical shape I'd been in my whole adult life. I felt energized, healthy and definitely not sick.

A close friend had sent me the article, which had prompted me to do a little investigating on the internet. While I was poring over other websites about various physical problems female runners had experienced, I noticed the word cancer kept appearing on the screen.

As I continued to read, the symptoms described were very similar to mine. This type of cancer is largely asymptomatic and is considered non-invasive. It's not like there's a lump in there that you can feel. Although I was more concerned than I'd previously been, I decided I wouldn't let my overactive imagination take over. Contradicting myself, I did make a decision to visit my gynaecologist; an appointment was made.

The following week, I was sitting in the doctor's office, feeling rather apprehensive while I waited to be called. I'd been a patient at this clinic for almost fifteen years. My doctor had delivered all three of my daughters and been through the various other ups and downs in my life. He'd have an answer, I confidently thought. After my name was finally called, I found myself sitting in his office explaining what had been happening over the past couple of months.

My last mammogram had been taken less than a year prior to this visit, but he suggested I have another one just to rule anything out. Maybe it was because of my age, I thought, as I'd recently turned forty-five. Perhaps it was because I was in good shape; whatever the cause, the doctor was confident it was nothing to worry about. He'd wait for the results of the mammogram and in the meantime advised me to go out and buy a more supportive bra; so my 'girls' wouldn't jiggle about as much when I was running. The bleeding, which wasn't constant or even annoying, should soon stop, he told me. I invested in a supportive running bra and, sure enough, the bleeding did stop. The results of my mammogram soon arrived and everything looked fine and my life carried on as normal.

However, just one month later, the bleeding had started again. This time it was heavier, particularly when I wasn't wearing a bra. After another visit to my doctor, I was sent to a special breast clinic. There I was given a laser imagery test and an ultrasound. Both tests confirmed the inevitable. I had cancer. The rest of that day was a complete blur. Everything seemed to speed up and get crazy. I was booked for a lumpectomy at the hospital just two weeks later; I was lucky and managed to get a cancellation. The operation went very well and the recovery was easy. I assumed my next visit to my oncologist would be my last. My brief encounter with cancer was done. Life would go on. Not so fast, Andrea: this would turn out not to be the case.

My next appointment with my oncologist would prove to be the most devastating. Not only was the lumpectomy unsuccessful at removing all the cancer, but suddenly I had all these older family members coming out of the woodwork with their depressing tales of breast cancer; what an experience!

Now I had to make a decision between another lumpectomy, where the doctors would try to get clean margins this time, or a full mastectomy. Not all women make such drastic choices. But, given my newfound family history, and knowing I'd worry for the rest of my life about the cancer coming back, I decided to have a double mastectomy. I'd also have an immediate reconstruction using tissue taken from my stomach.

Through this journey, my running had taken on even more importance. I was now running for my life. Running gave me purpose, refreshed my mind and reminded me I was alive. I even made race plans in order to keep training with a purpose and my mind focused. I ran most days up until the very day I entered the hospital for the biggest operation of my life. It was a lovely run and I remember it well; but not because it would be a while before I laced up my running shoes again.

It was a warm summer evening on 2 August when I was admitted to the hospital for my operation. I felt so alone in the hospital room that night and had a multitude of worrying thoughts racing through my mind. I had fought and pushed to have surgery as soon as possible. In some ways, I was relieved.

This would be the end of the cancer. They would get it all out and I would be on the road to recovery. I'd have probably seen the whole night round, if it wasn't for the medication they administered to help me sleep.

I was woken and out of bed early the next morning. I was going into theatre at 8:00 A.M. I had two surgical teams waiting for me. One was led by my oncologist, who would be doing the mastectomies. He estimated that the operation would take around three and a half hours. The next team would be led by the plastic surgeon who would do the reconstruction. It transpired this part of the operation took a massive seven hours. When I came out of recovery, the whole day had come and gone, and it was now dark outside.

During my last appointment with my plastic surgeon before surgery, I was told I'd feel like I had been run over by a truck when I woke from the operation. You may think this was a silly thing to say, but it actually helped me prepare mentally. Not that I know what it's like to be run over by a truck, but I remember thinking, when I woke up in my hospital room, this must definitely feel worse than being hit by a truck. I had drains coming out of both sides of my chest and two others coming out of my pelvic area. My legs were covered in what looked like 'space boots', which expanded and contracted in order to prevent blood clots from forming in my motionless legs. I had two more blood transfusions on top of the two units they gave me during surgery. I was too weak to have a port installed for pain medication. They therefore had to administer it through injections every few hours. Yes... it really was like I'd been run over by a truck, I can assure you. Luckily, thanks to the anaesthetic, that first night was a blur. The adult members of my family were all there when I was brought out of theatre; what a sight I must have been. For some reason, I was placed on the maternity ward to recover. The weather had suddenly turned very humid and the room, which had no air conditioning, was stifling hot. I kept drifting in and out of sleep as they watched over me.

I was in hospital for six days. My mum and sister, who are both practising nurses, spent the entire day during my hospital stay with me. They made sure I was washed and was moved in bed and later helped me get up.

By the time I was discharged, I really did feel ready to leave. Looking back, I was still quite weak. Thankfully, my parents lived with me for the six weeks after I was discharged. This certainly helped and increased the speed of my recovery. I couldn't walk up or down stairs and wasn't allowed to walk outside on my own. The doctors were worried that, if I fell, it would have a detrimental effect on my whole healing process. I was also not allowed to drive.

During this time of recovery, I did a lot of thinking. Going through cancer is a life-changing experience. I'm sure most cancer survivors will tell you the same thing. I wasn't the same after I'd gone through the operations and follow-up treatment. I did much soul searching. I found out who my true friends were and who truly loved me. I can now distinguish between the positive people and influences in my life and those who aren't.

Four weeks into my recovery, I received my pathology results. The supposed slow-moving and non-invasive cancer had started to migrate through my lymph nodes. As a result, they took seventeen of my nodes out on the side the cancer had been lurking. So this wasn't the end after all. I was sent to another hospital, to what they call a 'Tumour Board'. There, a team of doctors including pathologists, oncologists and other cancer specialists met and discussed my case. They collectively decided what they felt would be the best approach for my treatment. The consensus was to prescribe eight rounds of chemotherapy. The doctor said to look at it as an insurance policy; that I was putting the optimum number of years of survival on my side. I'll never forget that day. Like the day I found out I had cancer, this day also passed like a slow-moving dream. I questioned myself over and over again; I wondered if this was even real. Was this really happening to me?

I was introduced to the oncologist who would be responsible for my chemotherapy. I was also introduced to my pivot nurse, or personal nurse, who would oversee my treatment. My 'new' oncologist gave me what for him must have been the millionth repetition of a speech on what tests I would undergo before starting the chemotherapy. He also went through the dangers of undergoing such severe treatment and explained what medication I would need to take during my treatment and why. Then, without asking, he took out a form and enquired if I was employed. He started filling it in while I nodded, confirming I had a job.

Herein lay what would be one of the forks in the road that I went down. I had a choice. I could have nine months off work with the stroke of a pen while I went through treatment and recovery. Yet I had no intention of stopping work, so politely pushed his completed form back to him, while explaining I wanted to continue working if I could; I tried to sound as confident as I could. I felt empowered when I told him and I truly believed it. It was the first post-operative decision I made that was in my best interest. I needed to prove to my daughters, who were thirteen, ten and seven years old, that I was going to be fine. I wanted to give a positive example of how someone can fight with strength and dignity. I wanted my family to have as normal a life as humanly possible. So I worked my sixty-hours-a-week job, except for the two days I needed to take off every second week for my treatment. I arranged to have my treatment on a Thursday, so that by Monday I had gone through my physical and mental crash and was back on track. Once you go through the first treatment, the others tend to keep the same pattern. It's like a rollercoaster ride with the same peaks and troughs each time you go around.

Some of the best advice I got at this stage of my journey was to bring a friend or family member to chemotherapy with me. I did as suggested and it made each session much easier for me to handle. We would spend the time together chatting, laughing and reminiscing; this really distracted me from the treatment. In my case, the toughest part of the treatment was actually at the beginning of each session, when they inserted the needle. It was always so hard for them to find a vein big enough. The stress for me was them being able to hook me up. Once that was connected, it was just a question of getting the prescribed drugs inside me.

Soon after the first chemotherapy treatment, the inevitable happened. My hair started to fall out. At first it was in tiny wisps but eventually it was coming out in bigger clumps. Fortunately, my hairdresser is also my friend. So, armed with my new wig, I went over to my friend Dianne's house to get my head shaved. This was another choice I wanted to make, and I'm so glad I made the decision. As with any opportunity I chose, it was empowering and allowed me to remain in control. I'd been mentally preparing for this since my personal nurse told me I'd lose my hair. I actually think it was harder on Dianne who was much more emotional over this than me. Once my hair was off, we made a cup of tea and looked at the wig. What were we to do with it? I stuck it on my head but it just didn't look right. It required a trim and needed to be much flatter. Eventually, we put the blow dryer on low and flattened the synthetic hair down. I knew it would take some getting used to, but it was the new 'me' – for at least six months anyway.

It's strange how much colder it is with no hair, but hair loss does have its perks. For a runner during the cold weather, you never get hat hair and taking a shower is less time consuming. You save on shampoo and other hair products, and towel drying your head is done in a matter of seconds. Beats the fifteen minutes it takes to blow dry. There's no such thing as a bad hair day, they're all the same. Just place the wig on your head and go. To be honest, the wig was the first thing to come off when I got home. The chemotherapy induced hot flushes, I felt so hot! I think the sight of my baldness was a little troubling to my pre-teen, so I'd wear a bandana to cover it up. I didn't wear the wig very much on weekends either. I wore it only on special social occasions or when going shopping with the girls.

Although I was somewhat sidelined by chemotherapy, it didn't keep me off the road and I ran as often as possible. I'm convinced that the effort to lace up my shoes actually gave me the energy to endure the treatment. I ran a five-kilometre race midway through my treatment and clocked one of my better times. I remember thinking to myself as I ran past the cheering spectators along the race route, 'Way to go, chemotherapy girl – you show them.'

The night before my last day of treatment, my three daughters and I made cupcakes for the nurses and doctors on the Oncology Ward. It was in part a celebration and a way to thank them at the same time. It provided hope for my daughters that they would have their mother back and that life would start to be normal again. We had a wonderful dinner that night with friends; it was the perfect tonic.

With the treatment officially over, it felt strange at first. I wasn't at the hospital being checked by my doctor and healthcare workers every two weeks. I didn't have the security of being able to ask questions whenever I wanted. It took a lot of getting used to not going to hospital. Initially, it felt like I'd just been dumped by a boyfriend, honestly. To celebrate this newfound freedom, and because my running was going so well, I made plans to run a half-marathon just four months after the end of my treatment. The belief I had in myself and my confidence in being able to finish the race were all I needed, even if I was a little bit slower than in my pre-cancer days.

My true transformation really began towards the end of the year. Breast cancer, or any cancer for that matter, places you in front of your greatest fear. I had a choice when looking that fear in the eye. I could laugh and believe in myself and my ability to survive or not. There was never a moment that

I didn't believe I'd get well. Even when I had my meltdowns while I was crashing off the steroids and medication following chemotherapy, my belief was still there. The transformation taking place now was more of me as a person. I had shed the previous skin I was wearing in my pre-cancer days and had become somehow different.

At first, it was the small things I noticed, like being more patient and more grateful for things like a beautiful moon, or the joy of hearing the waves while I walked along the beach. It's the appreciation of seeing the loving smile on my daughter's face as she sleepily gazes up at me upon awaking. Although these things may have given me joy before, I now noticed them more. I had a newfound tendency to see the glass half full. I no longer angrily shout at the car in front of me in rush-hour traffic, in my haste to get to work. I listen to inspirational CDs now, or sing along to a great song in the peace of my car instead. In fact, I sit quietly in amusement when someone I know loses it because something is making them angry.

Like tending a garden, I was transforming my life in other ways as well. Some of the friends I once had were replaced by others. It's not because we had a falling out, but because my needs had changed and my goals were no longer the same. Family members who were once irritating ceased to be that way. Not because they had changed, but because I was more open minded. I don't let things get to me as much as they once did. Perhaps it's a result of looking proverbial death in the face and winning.

I don't take life as seriously as I once did. I laugh more and like to linger more in the moment. I'm grateful for the little conversations I have and take time to say mental thanks for the people I have them with. Unlike a young child, I no longer wish time would speed ahead to that special day or celebration. I'm patient, knowing that day will come with many other pleasurable moments in between. When I'm invited somewhere, I go giving my full attention. I don't leave half my thoughts at the door because I'm too busy thinking of the lengthy to-do list waiting at home.

Material things are less important to me. It's more important to have a car that keeps me safe and runs well than to own a specific model. I would rather spend my money on travelling and creating memories than own a special piece of jewellery. I prefer to spend my money on hosting a nice meal at home for my friends or family and enjoying each other's company before, say, buying another television.

I treat my body with more respect and keep up with my exercise. My diet is much healthier and I'm much more conscious of what goes in my mouth. I have discovered the joy of cooking. Spending time in the kitchen is now another way I relieve stress. I love spending a few hours making a good meal and look forward to poring over my ever-increasing collection of cookbooks looking for new culinary inspirations. Wholesome and nutritious foods are much more prominent in my family's diet, and it gives me great pleasure that they are eating well. While in the kitchen I have a smile on my face and I'm at peace.

As a survivor, I have devoted part of my running to supporting races that help cancer charities. Those races are even more special to me and inspire me to think of a future where I'll spend more of my time helping other cancer patients. I have started this through my writing. A year ago, I started a blog; it's a survivor's look at breast cancer. I write about running for health, running for hope and running for a life without breast cancer. This blog is not only therapeutic to me, but it's also my way of helping cancer patients who are now having treatment I once had. My hope is to inspire and perhaps just show them that, as with life in general, there is always a choice.

I'm at a point in my life where I am still growing.

The transformation into my new body is not yet complete. My journey has provided me with a life experience unlike any other.

I now know how powerful the mind is and how productive and successful we can be by properly exercising our thought process. The stories in this book will attest that everyone has the ability to be tenacious.

In life we have choices; the only question is whether we are ready or strong enough to seize the opportunity when it presents itself. My wish is to provide that inspiration. Cancer has been a massive life-changing experience for the better, but you shouldn't have to be diagnosed with cancer in order to realize this. Things happen for a reason and this is mine. It is also my gift back to you.

MAD DOGS AND ENGLISHMEN

MEMBERSHIP: # 1

What is it with our obsession to rush down the beach the moment the sun shines? I'm not moaning – at least we're getting a summer this year.

Like stranded seals on a beach, and as regular as salmon swimming upstream to mate each year, we wallow in the sand frying our skin that hasn't seen daylight since this time last year.

Men lie there motionless, fighting a losing battle to hold in their stomachs, while adamantly refusing to use coconut-scented suntan lotion. Women slowly slip into swimsuits, using as much care as a bomb disposal expert, desperate to ensure their towels don't hit the floor before their tops are securely fastened. Men watch under the camouflage of their sunglasses, hoping to see flesh that's normally only displayed on the top shelf of a newsagent.

So it's no wonder skin cancer has quadrupled over the last thirty years. There are two main types of skin cancer: non-melanoma, which is very common, and malignant melanoma, which is less common but more serious. It's estimated there are over 100,000 cases of non-melanoma skin cancer in the UK each year. Over the last twenty-five years, rates of malignant melanoma in Britain have risen faster than any other common cancer.

While women lie on a beach covering themselves in every combination of lotion they can find, as if replicating the mating habits of a peacock, men, on the other hand, prefer to burn like bacon in a frying pan, thinking it's a sign of weakness to use any sun protection.

This is proven in the statistics; men are more likely to develop a malignant melanoma, normally found on their chest or back, and women on their legs.

Nearing the end of the day, the guys' attention moves from the bronzing bodies around them to the forthcoming BBQ, an extravagant purchase that was acquired along with the oscillating fan and new garden furniture from a retail outlet earlier in the year. All purchased in hope of showing off to neighbours and proving to the women that we men can be spontaneous.

Although non-melanoma skin cancer is extremely common, in the vast majority of cases if detected early it's not life-threatening. Survival rates have been improving for the last twenty-five years and are now among the highest for any cancer. The latest malignant melanoma survival rates show that over eighty percent of men and around ninety percent of women survive the disease for at least five years after diagnosis.

While the men now stand impatiently waiting, shocked that their wives' faces now look like the skin shed from a snake, their wives give impressions of escapologists as they prise themselves out of their beachwear, their limbs feeling as taut as drum skins, and pulling faces like a tortoise eating lettuce.

So the moral of this column, should you not have got the subtle message by now: the next time the clouds drift away and you get the urge to lie and relax in the sun... Use some sunscreen...

LIVE LIFE TO THE FULL

MEMBERSHIP: # 11

Everything was going so well in my life, until finding a lump in my collar bone. I had a routine smear test scheduled for March so decided I'd mention the lump to the nurse at the same time. I hoped if nothing else it would put my mind at rest. I was twenty-nine years old and foolishly thought nasty things only happened to older people, which helped dismiss my fears. When the nurse said it wasn't anything to worry about, I felt a bit stupid for even mentioning it. I went home pleased my smear test was over and relieved my lump hadn't been anything to worry about either.

I'll be honest, I paid little attention to it from then on, even though it was gradually getting bigger. During April, I happened to mention it to my mum. She suggested I go and see my doctor and get it checked again, advice I stupidly ignored. After a couple more weeks of Mum nagging me,

I eventually booked an appointment with my doctor. The doctor repeated what the nurse had told me; he too didn't think it was anything to dwell on. However, just as a precaution, he would arrange for an ultrasound to be done. Before my ultrasound appointment, the doctor wanted me to have some blood tests done. These thankfully all came back as normal. Again, I wasn't the least bit concerned that there might be a problem.

The ultrasound was booked for 14 May. My sister came with me and it didn't take any time at all. While the ultrasound was taking place, I enquired what the lump could be. The lady said it looked like a swollen lymph node, and I thought nothing more of it.

She explained I'd receive a letter from the Ear, Nose and Throat (ENT) Department in about a week with the results. When I got home, I Googled 'lymph nodes' and the word cancer kept appearing everywhere; I was now starting to get quite worried.

My appointment for the ENT clinic arrived for 21 May. By now, I'd already convinced myself something nasty was going on. I imagined an invasion of bad cells crawling around my body, which I had no control over.

The 21st soon came round, and both Mum and Dad wanted to come with me, which I wasn't best pleased about. I'd already decided I wanted to go on my own. I went straight to the hospital from work in the end. I arrived at the department to see a waiting room full of people and was told all the day's appointments were delayed by about an hour.

Finally, at 5:00 P.M., I was called in to see the consultant. He said with a 'no messing' manner, 'I'm ninety percent sure you have cancer.' He went on to say he needed to take a biopsy to be sure, and to determine what type I had.

I couldn't believe what I was hearing. To think it might be cancer was one thing, but to actually hear what I did was something else. I stayed strong and managed not to cry – despite really wanting to. The consultant went on to explain that he required the biopsy as a matter of urgency so had actually already booked it for the following day. I was in complete shock by this stage; everything was suddenly happening so fast. I couldn't hold back my tears any longer and started to cry. I signed some paperwork and left the hospital. I was a complete mess, not knowing how I was going to drive myself home.

I called Mum and told her what the doctor had said, and she also started crying. It felt like I couldn't breathe, like I was being suffocated. All I wanted to do was curl up in bed and pretend it wasn't happening. This had to be a mistake, I kept saying to myself. Eventually, I managed to drive myself home, made a few phone calls and went to bed. But I couldn't sleep; I just lay awake all night going over and over what I'd been told. I kept wondering why it had happened to me. My whole life suddenly felt like it was collapsing around me.

I arrived at the hospital early the following day and was shown to my bed. I was in a room with three other ladies who were really nice and helped keep my spirits up. We chatted constantly for most of the day, which was a great help. Around 4:30 P.M., I was finally taken down to theatre. At about 6:00 P.M., I remember waking up and fussing around my neck to see if they'd put a drain in. I was so pleased when I found they hadn't. I had to stay in hospital overnight, which

I wasn't pleased about. Mum and Dad visited me, and they arrived just after I'd been taken back to the ward. Mum helped me put on my nightwear, as I couldn't move my neck or lift my arm properly; it was so painful.

The next day, the consultant came round, checked my stitches and signed me off work. He said I was now free to go home, but would have to come back a week later to have my stitches removed.

I returned to the ENT Clinic on 4 June. My consultant simply said, 'It's as we feared… you have cancer… we're sure its Hodgkin Lymphoma.'

It sounds a dumb thing to say, but I was ready to hear this news. I'd had nearly two weeks to get used to the idea and in truth the consultant had already told me before the biopsy was taken. There was no way he would have said he was ninety percent sure I had cancer if he wasn't. I left the hospital alone clutching various booklets on the subject.

Now I had to wait for my next appointment, which had already been booked for 12 June. I felt completely numb, scared and overwhelmed by the whole situation.

The date soon arrived; this was the appointment where I'd find out what treatment I needed. They'd also explain how long I'd be treated for and what stage cancer I had. Usually stages were described as numbers, between I and IV, which represented the amount that the cancer had spread. To my horror, I was a stage IV, this being the worst. The stage also takes into account the size of the tumour and how much it has invaded other organs. The consultant went through everything with me and made me feel a little more relaxed. I was told I would need a PET scan to see if the cancer had spread.

He wanted me to have it as soon as possible, to enable them to start treating me. I also needed my bone marrow tested; I wasn't looking forward to that.

I had a list of questions, which he answered, so it was just down to me to process and understand all the information I'd been given. I really didn't know where to start; all I wanted to do now was get the bone marrow test over with and find out if the cancer had spread. My consultant explained I'd need ABVD chemotherapy, but it would depend on the results from the PET scan. This would determine how much chemotherapy I needed, which would then be followed up with a course of radiotherapy.

My PET scan was booked for 19 June. I didn't really know what to expect but figured it was a pain-free procedure so couldn't be too bad. I was right; I had an injection, which contained a small amount of radiation. The radiation evidently sticks to the cancer cells, allowing the doctors to see how big the tumour is and if it's still active. I then had to wait a couple of hours for the radiation to work its way around my body before I could have the scan. I was in the actual scanner for about forty-five minutes and then went home.

I had to go back to hospital on 25 June for my bone marrow biopsy, which I was dreading. I arrived at the chemotherapy ward where I was shown to a bed. A doctor soon appeared and explained the procedure to me. He asked if I would like to be sedated or stay awake. I figured staying awake would be the best option, as I could go home the second it was over. How wrong I was – it was very uncomfortable. I thought I dealt with the pain quite well until the doctor said he wanted to take a second sample, as his first attempt had fallen out of the tool he was using. I soon decided I couldn't take the pain any more and got them to knock me out with a sedative. I obviously couldn't tell you what happened from there. I decided from that point on, if I was ever offered anything, it was being offered for a reason. Therefore, the answer I always gave from then on was yes. I never once tried to be brave again; I don't do pain.

My first dose of chemotherapy was on 3 July. I arrived on the ward and had to wait an hour for the drugs to arrive. One of the nurses put a line in the back of my hand to give the chemotherapy through. The nurses were lovely and I met another girl with the same problem as me. She was on her third lot of chemotherapy and we got on well straight away. My treatment arrived and it took around two hours for it to slowly drip down the clear tube and into my body. I didn't feel a thing and went home quite happy.

I expected to start feeling poorly that night but didn't, to my relief. I can honestly say I just felt warm and had a rather flushed face. This was on the Friday and I continued to feel OK over the weekend and Monday. However, Tuesday wasn't such a good day. I woke up with a really sore mouth; it was so sore that I couldn't eat anything as it hurt too much. I called the hospital who gave me a mouthwash, which helped straight away and I soon started to feel well again.

On Wednesday, I was feeling poorly again. My left arm, which I was given the chemotherapy in, had become very painful and swollen. I called the hospital and they suspected I might be reacting to one of the drugs. They suggested I put some heat on my arm; this would help the small veins remain open and should relieve the pain. The next day, one of the nurses called me to see how I was doing. There wasn't any improvement so I went back to the hospital to see a doctor. They confirmed I had reacted to one of the stronger drugs and all they could do was prescribe some painkillers. The pills actually made me feel sick so I soon stopped taking them. However, they were right: keeping heat on my arm did help with the pain. I couldn't go to work so sat in front of the television with a hot water bottle on my arm. I must have looked mad doing this in the middle of summer.

The day of my second chemotherapy session soon arrived. I had some blood tests done first thing and then had to wait to see the consultant. He confirmed I was well enough to have my second lot of chemotherapy. So reluctantly I went upstairs to the ward, to find out how long it would be before my drugs were available. The doctors had also decided they were going to fit me with a PICC line, to avoid the situation with my arm hurting again. One of the nurses fitted the line, which wasn't that painful, and I then had an x-ray, just to check the PICC line had been positioned correctly, before it was used. Thankfully, the line was working perfectly and my treatment could go ahead.

I sailed through this next lot of treatment and had no problems with my arm or with my mouth. I wasn't even sick this time so was feeling much happier. This meant my first cycle was out of the way. I only needed two more before I could find out if the cancer invasion to my body had stopped.

Sadly, two weeks after having my first lot of chemotherapy, my hair slowly started to fall out. I had always said, as soon as it began to fall out, I'd shave it all off, but actually I wasn't brave enough. This really upset me and I couldn't get my head round the fact that I had cancer. Cancer was something that happened to other people, not me. The nurses kept saying I should have my hair cut short as it lasts longer, but I didn't see the point. I didn't want to have my long hair cut before, so why would I now? There were advantages – I didn't need to shave my legs and my bikini line needed little attention.

I had always said that I wasn't going to wear a wig but my attitude towards them changed. I went to the hospital to pick my free NHS wig, but they didn't have the one I wanted, so I ended up with a wig I wasn't completely convinced about. I soon decided I wasn't going to wear it, so went shopping with Mum to find some headscarves. I was in a local shop speaking to a very kind lady, casually picking loads of different scarves, when a wig on a stand caught my eye. I tried it on and immediately thought it was fabulous. I had no idea at the time what it cost, but I didn't care: this was the wig for me. As soon as I got home, I called my hairdresser. She shaved off my hair and sorted out the fringe on the wig. I still think my hair falling out was the worst and most upsetting part of the whole experience, however painless. Nothing actually prepared me for it, but once I'd got the wig I soon got used to the idea. When people saw me for the first time, they just assumed I'd had my hair cut differently, which I was obviously very pleased about.

My second cycle of chemotherapy was supposed to start on 31 July and I was actually feeling quite good about it. I went to see the consultant, who said I couldn't have any chemotherapy just yet, as my white blood cells hadn't recovered from the last cycle. White blood cells, or leukocytes as my doctors sometimes called them, are responsible for our immune system. They defend the body from infectious diseases; without them we'd soon get an infection and die. I obviously had mixed feelings about not having my next lot of chemotherapy, but there wasn't anything I could do about it. The consultant explained that I'd have to wait until next Friday before I could start the second cycle. In future, I would need to have white blood cell booster injections.

As Mum and Dad were with me and it was a lovely summer's day, we decided to go to the seaside. It was great to get some fresh air and be somewhere nobody knew I was ill. I played on the two-pence fruit machines and ate prawns, chips and candyfloss. For just a few hours I felt like me again; I felt the cancer bubble I'd been trapped in had temporarily burst.

My second cycle was now starting on 7 August. My white cells had recovered so I was ready for the chemotherapy. I had breakfast while waiting for the drugs to arrive, and some two hours later I'd had my treatment. However, that weekend I felt completely knocked out and all I did was sleep.

In fact, I slept for most of the time, right up until Thursday of the following week. I loved my bed and sleeping, but this was crazy. The only thing I needed to remember was the white cell boosting injections. I needed five of them, one every day from the fifth day after having the chemotherapy. The district nurse came round each day for the five days. This had really started to wear me down. I decided it would be easier if I gave myself the injections.

I had the last treatment of my second cycle on 21 August. I soon found the chemotherapy days were rolling round quickly and I was now over halfway. My blood tests came back good because of the booster injections, so I had yet more chemotherapy. When I got home, I felt knocked out again; sleep had quickly become my new best friend. Again I got off lightly; I wasn't sick at all and I had no other nasty side effects.

On the day of my first injections, I went to the hospital so they could teach me how to do it. I have to say it was very easy once I got over the initial bit of sticking a needle into my tummy. So everything was going well with my treatment and I had been feeling fine. In my mind, there was no reason why my third cycle should be any different. I had the chemotherapy and went home, but to my complete surprise I felt rather poorly on the Monday. I couldn't decide if I wanted to sleep or watch television. I wanted to be sick, very sick. I was soon introduced to my second best friend: the toilet. I spent hours with my head hung over the toilet – anything and everything triggered it. From drinking water, eating, taking pills, mouthwash to cleaning my teeth, you name it, it made me feel sick. My mouth became quite sore again and I kept going hot and cold, and when I say cold, I mean freezing. I didn't know what to do with myself, and nor did anyone else; I was in such a bad mood, too.

I was hoping 18 September would be the last time I'd do the dreaded chemotherapy trip to hospital. I hadn't felt great for the previous two weeks since my last treatment and to make things worse I was developing a cold. I visited my consultant, who gave me the bad news that I couldn't have any more chemotherapy, because of my cold.

He told me to come back on Monday and I would hopefully be able to start again. Monday arrived and my cold was even worse, so I couldn't have the chemotherapy yet again.

I'd have to wait until Friday now. By Friday, the cold had thankfully disappeared and I was feeling much better. I was ready to get the last lot over and done with. I was also a little apprehensive as I'd be having a scan to see if the cancer had gone. My chemotherapy finally went ahead and I went home pleased it was all over, yet concerned how I was going to react this time. Not very well was the answer. I thought I was sick a lot the first time, but that was nothing compared to how I was this time. I just wanted everything to end and I never wanted to have to do this again. I dreaded the thought of the scans coming back saying there were still signs of cancer lurking.

I arrived at the hospital on 9 October, feeling really apprehensive and more emotional than I'd ever felt. I had my blood tests as normal and then began the wait. A nurse called Joanne came to see me and explained they were just waiting for the pictures from the PET scan to be reviewed. She suggested I come back at noon when hopefully they'd have the results. Those three hours were the longest of my entire life. I went back to the hospital at exactly midday, hoping and praying for good news. Joanne came in and shouted across the room to me, 'No more chemotherapy.' I burst out crying. I was so happy, I'd beaten cancer. I went upstairs to have my PICC line removed and was told that they would be in touch about having the radiotherapy. I was now finally free.

I went straight home, changed and hit the shops for a new outfit. I had to go out to celebrate. I sent a text to all my friends and arranged a quiet drink down the pub. I was collected at 7:30 P.M. and when I walked into the pub all hell broke loose. My best friend Emma had arranged a surprise party for me. All my friends were there and I had the best time ever. I had presents, cards, a disco and lots of drinks. I didn't want it to end and it's something I will remember for the rest of my life.

I still had to have radiotherapy but I was told it would be a breeze compared to the chemotherapy, so I wasn't too worried about it. I had to have a mask made, which went over my head. It was basically to stop me moving on the table and to keep my chin out of the way. I didn't like the mask very much and was bolted to the table with it on. I had to have three weeks of radiotherapy, every day for five days a week. The first week was fine – in fact, it was a complete pain having to go to the hospital every day for less than five minutes' treatment. In week two, I started to feel a bit poorly; my mouth and throat were very sore and I lost my voice. My throat was so bad by the end of week two that I couldn't eat. I even struggled to drink water. I then began to dread every day as it made it worse. I actually ended up with two ear infections, a throat infection and one in my mouth. Due to not being able to eat or drink comfortably, I lost two stone in weight. I finally finished my last week of radiotherapy and was over the moon and prayed I'd never have to go there again. I had an appointment with the doctor and he assured me the infections were under control and my body would return to normal within a few weeks.

I've now been in remission for nearly four years. I have my next lot of scans booked for December just to make sure the cancer hasn't returned. Looking back, it was a very long, tough year, but in some ways I wouldn't change it. I have learnt a lot about what's important in life and what's not so important.

The doctors told me I should take it easy for a while; however, I soon went back to work full-time. I do get tired but it is nothing an early night can't fix. I appreciate more than ever that I've just one life, and I should live it to the full.

IF IN DOUBT, PERSEVERE

MEMBERSHIP: # 12

It was during January when I first thought something was wrong. I kept getting a feeling of immense pressure in my head, which increased each time I bent down. I'd never experienced this before so was naturally concerned. This, together with an irritating cough, finally prompted me to visit the doctor. Strangely, these symptoms always felt a lot worse at night.

My worries were soon put to rest when I was prescribed a spray for post-nasal drip. The doctor explained my symptoms were caused by my sinusitis, something I suffered with; I got this nearly every winter when I caught a cold.

Later that week, I started having problems breathing. I first noticed it while taking a physical education lesson at the primary school where I worked. I went to the doctor again, and this time he gave me a course of antibiotics as he thought I might possibly have a lung infection.

Over the next couple of weeks, my breathing continued to get worse. Even just a gentle stroll to the local shops caused a feeling of breathlessness. The feeling of pressure in my head also continued, which obviously worried me.

Yet again, I went back to my doctor. This time, I was referred to an Ear, Nose and Throat (ENT) specialist, as my doctor still thought my problems were linked to my sinus issues. I'd also noticed my neck had become swollen. I did actually wonder if I was imagining it as it appeared to come and go.

However, when I met up with a friend whom I hadn't seen for three weeks, she commented how puffy my cheeks looked.

I paid yet another visit to the doctor, as I'd now noticed the problem was only on my right side. The doctor thought I might have a problem with my thyroid this time, so suggested I have an ultrasound of my neck. Things soon came to a head at the end of February. I was having a wash and noticed a purple, spider-like pattern of veins under my breasts. At first I thought it was merely a side effect from where my bra had been digging in, due to my constant coughing recently.

I decided it was best to go and see the doctor again; this time, she suggested I have some blood tests. I was told there was no urgency, so booked the next available appointment, which was the following week.

Desperate for some answers when I got home that afternoon, I started surfing the internet. Instinctively, I knew when I found a condition called Superior Vena Cava Syndrome (SVCS), which stated the main symptom as 'a feeling of pressure in head and neck when bending forward', that I'd found what was wrong with me. When I continued to read, I recognized I had practically all the other symptoms, too. I was now becoming very worried, almost terrified when I saw that SVCS is caused by a form of cancer in most cases. I called my doctor straight away, and she said she'd see me immediately. The doctor didn't think my diagnosis was correct, because I was not having the classic symptom of severe morning headaches; however, to be on the safe side, she sent me to have a chest x-ray.

I was now a lot happier, having seen the doctor, probably because I felt I'd made a wrong diagnosis and was hopefully closer to finding out what was wrong with me.

The next day, I received a call asking if I could go and have a CT scan first thing the following day. This raised my suspicions that perhaps I did have something wrong with me after all. I managed to take my mind off the scan by keeping myself busy – the house had never looked so clean. Everyone kept saying I shouldn't believe everything I read on the internet.

First thing the next morning, I went off to the hospital for the scan. That evening, the doctor phoned me at home and told me it was bad news. She said they'd found a tumour pressing on my Superior Vena Cava Vein, which is the main vein that carries blood to the upper body and lungs. So, unfortunately, my own self-diagnosis had been right.

The next day, the doctor had arranged for me to see an oncologist at my local hospital. Thankfully, I'd got the first appointment of the day. It was at this appointment they confirmed I had SVCS. I was told that they were unsure if I had lung cancer or lymphoma. The oncologist arranged for me to have various other tests including a bronchoscopy.

At the beginning of March, I went back to the hospital for a CT-guided lung biopsy. I had to stay in hospital for a few hours afterwards to recover. The following week, I was due to hear the results, and needless to say the night before wasn't easy – more cleaning.

When I saw the doctor, she started asking me yet more questions and wanted to examine me. The suspense was killing me. 'What have I got?' I asked.

My doctor looked up and replied, 'Quite honestly, I don't know.'

The tests were inconclusive so the biopsy sample needed to be retested. The doctor explained that cells from both lymphoma and lung cancer look very similar when examined under a microscope. She said that full recovery from either was possible, but the chances would be much greater if I had a type of lymphoma. She went on to talk about Non-Hodgkin (NHL) and Hodgkin Lymphomas in more detail, which made me hopeful that I had one of these and not lung cancer. The doctor said she'd phone me at home the moment she got the results. However, my husband rightly felt it would be much more beneficial if we were given the results face-to-face, and I agreed. The wait at home was difficult but I was becoming an expert at keeping busy. We found ourselves trying out a new juicer, which had been recommended by a work colleague of my husband. He coincidently at the time was fighting his own battle with lung cancer, which he has now won.

At 4:00 P.M., the phone rang; my heart was thumping as I answered it. The doctor said it was good news and there was no need to go back to the hospital that day. She told me that it was a type of NHL and explained that, as standard procedure, I'd need to have my bone marrow tested and some more blood tests. It's a strange thing to say that NHL was 'good news'.

The bone marrow test wasn't brilliant; it was very painful but I did my best to think about other things. I also had another CT scan. The next day, I met a consultant at the Christie Hospital and explained my story and symptoms to him. It was then I was diagnosed with primary Mediastinal large B-cell Lymphoma, which affects more women than men at a ratio of 9:1. Mediastinal Lymphoma is very difficult to diagnose unless a chest x-ray is taken, this is because there are normally no lumps that can be felt, and even listening through a stethoscope gives no definite clues.

I found this time unbearable; I just wanted to get on with my treatment and get rid of the cancer. I really deteriorated physically. I could hardly walk upstairs and any form of movement was pretty difficult. My cough by now had become really painful and I needed to rest my head on my pillow to help relieve the pressure. In addition to this, my upper body had also become very swollen and I found sleeping in a chair helped.

My treatment started on 31 March, twelve days after first being diagnosed. I got through it the best I could, reminding myself of my good prognosis. It was a long process, however, and I had all the normal side effects after each dose of chemotherapy. This made me feel like I was coming down with flu or had drunk too much alcohol; I wish. I also felt nauseous, but the anti-sickness medication really helped a lot. I had six cycles of a chemotherapy regime called R-CHOP, each dose three weeks apart. I made it my target to help myself as much as I possibly could. I rested when necessary, especially during the first week. I changed my diet to include more fruit and vegetables. Juicing had become a way of life, eliminating most refined sugars where possible.

I really enjoyed having visitors when in hospital but I made sure I only saw them when I was feeling OK. I managed to avoid picking up any infections but I did get shingles twice. This is common during treatment but both times I acted quickly and was given the anti-viral drug Aciclovir, which was really effective.

At the end of August, I had a PET scan, which showed that my tumour had reduced from about 9 cm to 3 cm in size. I then had some fifteen sessions of radiotherapy to eradicate this. By the middle of September, I had finally completed the treatment.

I was lucky enough to have had tremendous emotional and practical support from both my family and friends. My husband was absolutely wonderful; I couldn't have managed without him. I also had reflexology treatments and post-treatment relaxation classes at a local hospice. Thankfully, the NHS reacted quickly once my diagnosis had been made. I was very glad that I followed my instincts to keep returning to my doctor and investigated my symptoms myself. I now know that Mediastinal Lymphoma is difficult to diagnose and I underestimated just how long it would take to regain my strength.

I decided to stop work during my treatment as I worked with children and didn't have the energy needed, especially as the treatment had sent me into an early menopause; but that's another story.

Now I'm doing some voluntary work, which I get a lot of satisfaction from. Although it sounds a cliché, I feel like a different person and I'm determined to make the most of the rest of my life. I feel so lucky to have found something I enjoy and appreciate every day.

I recently received the results of my latest PET scan, almost a year to the day since my first session of chemotherapy.

My consultant is very pleased with the results, so I just need regular check-ups now. I'll be continually monitored for the next ten years.

Since my experience with cancer, I have travelled quite a bit, done a lot of voluntary work and have pursued my desire to write poetry – all things I'd have never done before.

HOW TO SOLVE A PROBLEM LIKE MY REAR

MEMBERSHIP: # 13

This is a story that may well sound disturbingly familiar in parts. For me, the scariest thing about being diagnosed with bowel cancer was not knowing I actually had anything wrong. My story starts on a typical day after work, with a few cold beers and a Chinese takeaway.

At the age of thirty-one, the world was my oyster, or so I thought. I had a lovely girlfriend called Rachel. I owned a small sales company and lived in a cracking apartment near Islington in North London; life was good. I was a bit of a workaholic, which led to a less than perfect lifestyle. Twelve-hour days were normal and most nights involved a couple of pints and a takeaway. Admittedly not ideal, but I was only thirty-one and allergic to cooking.

Around midnight one Saturday after an evening of drinks with colleagues, I went home clutching my favourite Chinese dish, Singapore noodles. These noodles tend to be rather spicy and had me rushing to the bathroom afterwards. No surprise there; I'm sure most of us have been in that situation before, so I thought nothing of it.

Monday morning arrived and I decided I'd throw a sickie. I'd had little sleep and my mysterious tummy rumblings had continued. I thought a quick visit to my doctor would be worthwhile, to see if perhaps I had an ulcer or something that needed treating. I did my best to describe to the doctor how I felt and said I now know what it's like to have period pains; she didn't laugh. Yes, I confirmed, I had felt quite tired lately, but work was really busy.

Yes, I confirmed again, there was a little blood on the toilet paper, but nothing unusual as I'd used it a lot recently. I felt like a fraudster as I didn't actually feel that ill by the time I got to see her. I left feeling like I shouldn't have wasted her time.

A couple of weeks later, I received a letter inviting me to see a consultant in hospital. This was not a great surprise, as my doctor had explained she'd refer me.

I attended the appointment as, at worst, it was another half day off work. The consultant was very nice and I relayed my tale of woe to her before she took her revenge, by digitally examining me. If a doctor says they are going to perform a digital examination, be warned it's not digital as in hi-tech, it's their finger digit.

With that over, I went back to work and thought nothing more of it. I was told it would be a couple of weeks before I got the results. Therefore, I completely forgot about dodgy takeaways, doctors and digital examinations. Although I'd forgotten, they hadn't. Another appointment letter soon arrived, requesting I have both a colonoscopy and CT scan. I attended unaware of the exact nature of a colonoscopy. This was an investigative procedure where a camera was inserted into my rectum and pushed into my colon. This without doubt is one of the weirdest feelings I've ever had.

The CT scan was a breeze by comparison. I simply had to drink some orange liquid that would show up on the scan. Then I was asked to lie down on a sliding table, which moved through a large, metallic-looking doughnut; simple. I felt strangely violated by all these tests. I was assuming by now that I had the mother of all ulcers or Irritable Bowel Syndrome (IBS).

On the evening before the results, I received a call from my mum asking if I wanted her to stay with me. Now I don't know about your parents, but, when my mum asks for something, it generally means it is going to happen – whether I want it to or not. I mentioned the fact that I was the managing director of my own company; I mentioned I was thirty-one; I also mentioned the fact that I'd been going to the doctors 'all by myself' for a very long time. Mum mentioned the fact that she was still my mum and she would see me at Euston train station later that day. It's nice to be asked though!

So, with Mum for company, we made our way from the train station to the hospital. I registered at reception and we sat down and waited to be called. I wasn't worried – I was still convinced I was pretty much OK, so was chatting with Mum about her developments at work.

Soon, I heard my name called; we stopped talking and looked up. I glanced at Mum and she sat down again saying, 'I'll wait here then.' I smiled and said I thought I could cope.

Once I'd knocked on the door, I walked in to see there were two other people with the doctor. One evidently was a junior doctor and the other I was told was the hospital registrar.

'Please take a seat, Mr Davies,' the registrar said.

Once the introductions were over, I sat down and couldn't help but ask, 'So, what's up, Doc?' while smiling insanely.

'You have adenocarcinoma of the colorectal region,' he replied.

'What's that?' I asked, my smile suddenly replaced with concern.

'You have cancer, Mr Davies.'

Now I appreciate at this point that we would all react in different ways, none better or worse, it's just who we are. I was a manager of a sales company and my mind went into problem-solving mode so I replied, 'Oh, OK, so what are we going to do about it?'

I just wanted to understand how to go from having to not having. Dying didn't even enter my mind. I didn't panic, cry, freak or hear 'Greensleeves' in the background; I was completely calm. I could tell my reaction shocked them a bit.

One thing I couldn't do though was tell Mum; I mean, what do you say? 'Hey, the good news is it's not an ulcer...'

The registrar said she'd tell her. Mum just replied, 'I thought so.' Could have told me, I thought.

They arranged a second appointment within two days, this time with the surgeon who would discuss my treatment options. The hardest thing was not being told I had cancer, but telling those who cared about me. Mum already knew, but I had to tell Rachel, Dad and other friends. I had mentioned to the guys at work that I'd probably be a bit late the next day. I arrived at the office once the morning meeting was over, around midday. It's a strange thing being told that you have cancer. Although you are officially ill, you don't have anything to show for it.

I was no more physically ill than the day before. In order to convince people that you are ill, you really need some visual evidence – coughing, sweating or your arm in a sling. However, because I had none of these things, interacting with people was a little disconcerting. They don't have anything to focus their attention on, no cast to write on or tissues to offer. It's a bit of a non-event and no one wants to ask you how you feel as it's a daft question in their minds; even if I was OK, which I was. So I sat down with a couple of the people closest to me and told them what I knew, which to be honest wasn't that much. I had cancer, it was not good and I had no idea what was going to happen until after the next appointment. One of my main concerns was what I was going to do workwise. Obviously, if I did die, it wouldn't be a major problem; however, as I was convinced that I wasn't going to 'shuffle off this mortal coil' just yet, I needed to start thinking about my short-term future. What was I going to do with the company? How was I going to survive financially, self-employed with no sick pay?

First things first, though – it was time to see the surgeon for my treatment options.

Rachel came to this appointment with me, as she wanted to get the real information not the second-hand version from me; again, I had no choice in the matter. Entering the room, we shook hands with the registrar and I was introduced to the consultant surgeon. He was an extremely friendly guy and made us both feel relaxed almost immediately. I explained that I was aware of the seriousness of the situation, but wanted to get on to the 'what's the solution and what can we do about it' part. I wanted to feel some level of control while in a fairly uncontrollable, very stressful position. The surgeon understood and we got down to business.

'The preferred method of dealing with cancer of the colon and rectum is surgery,' he explained. 'Fifty years ago, a surgical technique was developed called an abdomino-perineal excision of the rectum.'

I raised an eyebrow at him; this was no time for big words.

I looked over at Rachel and gave her a reassuring thumbs up – fifty years ago, no problem, I thought.

He continued, 'It's a fairly major operation, which is designed to completely remove the threat of cancer from the area.'

'Sounds good,' I agreed. 'So what does the procedure involve?' I was feeling pretty optimistic – *completely remove the threat of cancer – cool.*

The surgeon then described the whole operation to both Rachel and myself. 'An incision is made from around your diaphragm all the way down to the base of your stomach,' he explained, while trailing a finger down my front to just below my beltline for added effect.

'Once you are opened up, we will go in through your stomach, take out your insides to get to the large bowel – obviously they will be replaced after the procedure is completed. Then we'll remove your entire large bowel and your anus.'

'What do you mean by remove my anus?' I felt that nugget of information needed further investigation.

'Well, it is like an apple core. To be on the safe side, we feel it's advisable to remove all possible areas where the cancer might spread to. So the large bowel and the anus are removed and where your anus was we would simply sew it together.' He reiterated with a twisting hand action to emphasize the apple core motion, just in case I hadn't got it completely the first time.

'OK, so this was fifty years ago – what new-fangled operation have we got now?' I knew that I was on to a loser here, but worth a try.

'I'm afraid that is it. There are other complications that you should be aware of, though.'

'Such as?'

'Going in through the stomach does bring us into close proximity to your genital region, and there is a chance of infertility.'

'That should return to normal, however!' chipped in the consultant.

'Indeed,' agreed the surgeon. 'However, there is another potential problem in that area. Running from your genitals up towards your stomach are a couple of nerves that control your erection. The surgery will be very close to these nerves and there is a chance that they might be damaged, which would therefore lead to permanent impotency.'

'What sort of chance?' I asked.

'About thirty percent, i.e. one in three.'

'You've never been in sales, have you?'

'Err, no!'

'Don't give up the day job,' I said. 'That was the worst pitch I've ever heard!'

'I'll bear that in mind.' She smiled.

'So you're telling me that, although in the last fifty years we've sent men to the moon, invented the internet and developed computers that can fit on the head of a pin, the best you can offer me is to remove my sodding arse?'

'Well, yes. If we are to be certain of getting all of the cancer, I can only recommend this procedure.'

'You'll have a colostomy bag, however, which is admittedly not the same but it is not as bad as you might imagine,' commented the consultant.

I just looked at her. This was not the kind of back-up plan I was expecting: a stoma or colostomy bag?

I don't think so. I appreciate that there are thousands of people who live full and rewarding lives after they have had a bag fitted.

'OK. So what would happen if I did nothing at all?' I asked.

'The tumour would continue to grow and eventually it would kill you,' replied the surgeon.

'How long would I have if I did nothing?'

'About twelve to eighteen months.'

So there we had it. In the space of two months, I'd gone from having an innocent takeaway and throwing a speculative sickie to having colorectal cancer and being offered what we like to call in the bowel cancer community the 'Bag or Box' option. I politely refused their kind offer and suggested they go back to the drawing board to find another option.

Owing to my requesting alternative solutions to the 'smash and grab' attempt on my arse, I'd been sent details of my personal chemotherapy and radiography timetable. This, however, was all about to change.

A couple of weeks after my diagnosis, Mum was having a coffee with a friend, and talking about my situation. Apparently, her friend's neighbour was an oncologist. In addition to this spooky coincidence, the oncologist and the surgeon specialized in – wait for it – colorectal cancers. He happened also to be the only person in the country who used a special form of radiotherapy, called Papillon, which is applied directly to the tumour. This could enable the surgeon to try an alternative micro-surgery, which would negate the need to remove my anus.

I was obviously stunned; I couldn't believe it. If ever something was meant to be, this was it. Within three days, the first appointment was made.

I didn't know if this was going to be the answer, as the doctors might not have been able to operate owing to the tumour's proximity to the muscle tissue of my sphincter. I had a feeling, though, that this was fate throwing its hat into the ring and I was just going to have to see how far it would take me.

Papillon was really designed for polyps and early-stage tumours and I had a T3a tumour, which was far too big for the Papillon and the micro-surgery called Transanal Endoscopic Micro-surgery (TEM). I had asked the original surgeon why we couldn't just shrink it and use the hole already there instead of ripping me apart and removing everything. 'We don't do that' was his reply.

Well, with twenty-five sessions of external beam radio-therapy running in conjunction with 5FU chemotherapy feeding continuously into my system via an arm-mounted infuser for ten weeks, that's exactly what we did. This traditional treatment was rough and my side effects were varied. Luckily, my hair didn't fall out, but the radiotherapy caused me pain like I've never felt before or since.

After the initial barrage, I had another MRI scan to assess its progress before discovering, after months of pain and anguish, if I would even qualify for Papillon and the TEM procedures. To my surprise and great relief, it had worked perfectly. Even without the next stages, the tumour had all but gone. This was great but also annoying as this was not new technology, just standard treatments that had all but nuked a T3 tumour. I had been left in no doubt that the only way forward was to perform radical and life-altering surgery. I wonder how many people simply go with their first diagnosis through fear of cancer and don't look for alternatives.

I had two sessions of Papillon, with a two-week break in between. The second as an out-patient only took a couple of minutes and some bowel preparation to perform it. It worked perfectly, and with the tumour all but gone I was told that I could go forward for the TEM, which would be performed two months later.

Papillon is effective because it delivers high doses of x-rays directly onto the tumour, at a very low power – oh, and some interesting positions. This means that after only a few millimetres the radiation levels are minimal with only the tumour taking the full impact, leaving healthy tissue alone.

I had my surgery on 30 January and have just passed my eight-year all clear, which in cancer terms means that I'm cancer free. I was only in hospital for a total of five days – two days before the operation eating mostly jelly and a couple after to check my normal bowel movements had returned. I pointed out that this was unlikely as I hadn't eaten anything for days and my arse was still in shock after having a three-inch hole cut out of it, but rules are rules. I had no temporary stoma and, apart from a slight problem with my back in the first few weeks afterwards, I was all good. Well, that's not totally true. Taking into account the hectic radiotherapy and chemotherapy regimes I had endured, and the hole in my colon, I never really had major physical problems. I had some skin reaction to extreme sun, part of the reason why I moved back to Manchester as I knew it wouldn't be an issue there. I still make sure I know where the toilets are whenever I go anywhere, but really I am physically in a far better place than I was before I had cancer.

However, as time went by, I was aware that something was wrong. Surely I should be looking at the world through rose-tinted glasses now that I had survived. I found, however, that in London I was getting increasingly angry at the way people treated each other. I found myself getting more and more impatient and frustrated with people. This was making me an angry person and to some degree it still does.

This is not who I am or who I wanted to be. As neither Rachel nor I was actually from London, we decided we should look at work options outside of the M25. I was soon offered a great job in Manchester, so we moved back up north, to be closer to my family and hospital, as I was still going for regular check-ups. Unfortunately, after a while, I realized that all was not well with the company. This led to an environment of fear and bullying with members of staff having to leave due to depression because of how they were being treated. If this was the real world, I didn't want to be part of it. My empathy for others had evidently increased during my illness, probably due to the suffering – and strength in battling it – that I witnessed every day in the cancer wards.

I would become angry for no reason or end up crying at *X Factor* when an unknown would sing like an angel and I could see how their life would never be the same again. I was an emotional wreck really but I had no idea what was happening to me. I had survived so I must be happy – surely? I tried once more to ignore that I had changed. I so wanted to be the same as everyone else. I just wanted to be 'normal' and give Rachel the life that she deserved. I wanted to be happy and I thought being like everybody else would allow me to do that – get a job, get married, have kids. I wanted it so much that I proposed to Rachel while working for the company. Obviously, I loved her to bits and so this was a no-brainer. It was only over Christmas some four years later that I finally admitted to myself that I'd had cancer and needed to start to deal with it.

It took four years after finishing my treatment to confront what had happened and how it had really affected me. This obviously sounds like a very strange and possibly selfish thing to say. I found the social pressures or expectations of having survived cancer were intense. I should be more aware of life, a life where the grass was greener, the sky bluer and small furry animals would flock around my bedroom window every morning. I should be happy that I was still alive and should be training for a marathon straight away. The problem was that my landlord, the taxman and the rest of the world just sprang back into focus. They hadn't changed just because I'd been ill; I'd just been preoccupied.

Having cancer was a release for me. I'd been driving myself into the ground with work and couldn't see an end to my situation. The cancer, while shocking, brought everything into focus. Suddenly, the day-to-day stuff just didn't matter any more. Then there was the feeling of isolation. I'd been in hospital every day for months, being cared for in a place where people had shown concern. For the first time in my life I felt special. That changed the day the tumour was removed.

I went from lots of social interaction and support to being home alone without an income, or a group of people to talk with. At work I was goal-focused and always had routines and plans to achieve those goals.

This helped me take little steps and not focus too much on the end goal. The problem was that I had no idea that I would feel this way and so thought that I was broken somehow and tried to ignore it completely. How dare I be depressed when I was well and so much luckier than so many others? Then I had a turning point and decided to write my own story. I found this really helped me and I hope it will help others, too. I have never really looked back since.

Cancer is scary but not as scary as I had thought. The bravest people I have ever met were in cancer wards and they shamed me with their strength and humour on many occasions. More people live long and happy lives after having cancer than ever before, and those who don't go down fighting. It's just a shame that as a species we are at our best when things are at their worst.

Thank you for reading my story and I hope that you learnt something from my journey that may help you in yours. Take care and good luck.

I have to go now because I need a poo!

NEVER GIVE UP

MEMBERSHIP: # 14

It was a summer I will always remember. I spent long, lazy, sun-filled days doing fun things with my two boys, Cameron and Cullen. Picnics, bike rides, sleepovers and a two-week holiday in Majorca. We spent the time there swimming, walking, exploring and eating too much. I guess you could say life was pretty fabulous. My boys went back to school and my husband, James, and I got busy preparing our house for the long-awaited and meticulously planned two-storey extension. We cleared junk and emptied the garage of rubbish and old furniture. We continued working on the house at the weekends, but always made time for our boys and social life, too!

One morning in September, I woke and unusually for me didn't feel at all hungry. I just had a cuppa and prepared the boys' breakfast. My lack of appetite continued for a couple of weeks, until James eventually noticed I wasn't eating breakfast every day. His comments made me realize I wasn't eating too much at other mealtimes either. I'd lost a few pounds in weight, but wasn't feeling particularly stressed about it. I simply assumed it was related to all the work we were doing in preparation for the new house extension.

'Go and see the doctor,' James insisted.

So, reluctantly, I made an appointment. My doctor examined me and I explained my lack of appetite and feeling of fullness after even the tiniest meal. He prescribed Gaviscon and gave a possible diagnosis of dyspepsia, otherwise called an upset stomach or indigestion.

Two weeks later, and now with absolutely no appetite and increased weight loss, I went to see the doctor again. I'm five feet, nine inches; therefore, it was very noticeable that I now weighed just nine stone. This time he suggested I have an endoscopy. I had this done privately just a week later and there was no evidence of any blockage or obstruction. I was also now starting to experience some pain in my left side. As I'd mentioned this to my consultant prior to the endoscopy, he also arranged for me to have an ultrasound. At this point, I wasn't especially worried as the endoscopy had come back 'clear'.

James was worried, but I managed to persuade him to continue with his work trips to Dubai and Bangalore. Within the week, I got a date for my ultrasound in the post. As James was away, I asked my mum to come with me so I'd have some company. The sonographer squirted a cold lubricant onto my tummy and began to scan the area. I lay there for a while, thinking about day-to-day stuff like work, the boys and jobs I needed to do at home. Suddenly, I realized I'd been lying there for a lot longer than I'd expected. The sonographer had been taking a long time scanning my left side. I could just tell by her body language that there was something wrong.

'Is everything looking OK?' I asked weakly.

'I need to speak to your consultant, but your pain is definitely not in your head,' the sonographer replied.

This might sound silly now in hindsight, but at the time I was relieved as I'd started to worry I was imagining the pain. I found Mum, who was sitting in the waiting room, and told her they'd found something, but I didn't know what. I left the hospital feeling very uncertain of what lay ahead.

I just kept telling myself I was thirty-nine, not ninety-nine, and I'd be OK. Unfortunately, James was still away in Dubai, and looking back this was one of the worst days, as my carefree life had suddenly vanished.

I tried to sound upbeat on the telephone later that evening when James called for a chat; however, he sensed immediately that something was wrong. At that instant, I really started to feel scared. I had my mum, but I didn't have James to support me so I felt very lonely and the nights dragged on forever. It took James two days to get home. When he finally got back, we just hugged and cried but I somehow managed to stay inwardly strong. No amount of worrying would change the outcome.

My next test was a CT scan, which showed a mass on my pancreas. Then I had an MRI scan to establish the size and location and whether the tumour was operable or not. Sometimes the internet is a good thing, but in my case everything I read was doom and gloom, with very few pancreatic cancer survival stories. The pain had definitely worsened and I was experiencing incredible discomfort on my left side and through into my back. By now I'd lost over one and a half stone in weight and was barely sleeping.

I sat my boys down and told them the doctors had found a tumour.

'Is it cancer?' Cullen asked.

'We aren't sure yet but the doctors think it might be,' I replied.

'Will you die?'

'I could, but I'll do everything I can to get better,' I replied and I meant every word I said.

In late November, I was shopping with Mum, desperately trying to organize Christmas presents.

It was always my job and I was determined this year would be no different. When my mobile started ringing, I knew the outcome of this call could change my life, so answered it nervously. 'It's operable,' my consultant said. I shook in disbelief and felt very excited. A whole mix of emotions rushed through my body: 'It's operable' meant I actually had a chance.

I was admitted to hospital on 4 December. Within just four hours, I'd had most of my pancreas removed. The surgeons also took out my large and swollen spleen, and parts of my adrenal glands were removed, too. I stayed in the Intensive Care Unit (ICU) overnight and was then moved to the Surgical Acute Care Unit where I spent the next week. I had a catheter fitted for five days and a central line in my neck. The morphine was making me really high and causing me to itch and hallucinate. The painkillers had to be injected into my stomach daily, which I didn't like too much. Eventually, the morphine was reduced, although a little too quickly for my liking and I spent the day in the most horrendous pain; I couldn't even speak. Eventually, at midnight, my consultant insisted I was given a Patient Controlled Analgesic (PCA), as I was in so much pain; I didn't stop pressing the button!

On the doctor's ward round the following day, my drain was still full and cloudy. 'Once you are off this drip you can go home,' the doctor said.

That was all the incentive I needed. Within twenty-four hours, I no longer needed the morphine and started taking tablets instead. Finally, after eight days, with the drain still in place, I was allowed home.

Moving about during the first week was a struggle. The simplest tasks, which I'd always taken for granted, such as getting out of bed, sitting up and walking were difficult. I needed a wheelchair for the first few days.

On 16 December, I received my histology report. The tumour was malignant: a moderate to poorly differentiated adenocarcinoma of the pancreas tail. My chemotherapy treatment would start in January.

That year's Christmas didn't feel very Christmassy at all, with no tree and no decorations like we normally had. That weekend James and Cameron proceeded to transform our house with me directing from the sofa. We had a lovely Christmas despite how sore, tired and worried I felt. A few family members came round on Christmas Day and extended family on Boxing Day. We did the usual Christmas family things – played games, drank too much and had a lot of laughs, too. On New Year's Eve, James and I had some friends and family over. On the stroke of midnight, I hugged everyone, knowing that the New Year meant chemotherapy and more uncertainty.

My first chemotherapy session was fine; within three hours, I was eating lunch with James, and then we went shopping for a wardrobe for our newly completed bedroom. I continued with chemotherapy every week for the next six months, having one week in every four off. As the weeks went on, I began to feel worse and certainly less tolerant of the poison going into my body.

My fortieth birthday in February was a quiet one. I'd always planned a great big party, but this would have to wait.

Some weeks I felt poorly from the chemotherapy; others I'd feel fine. I had a total of eighteen sessions and marked each one off my calendar as I had it. I always looked at the end goal and remained positive throughout.

Thankfully, I didn't totally lose my hair, although it did thin considerably and eventually I made the heart-breaking decision to have my long hair cut into a shorter style.

Throughout my chemotherapy, I tried to stay as fit as possible and walked regularly as well as using the treadmill whenever I was strong enough. I signed up for the five-kilometre 'Race for Life' and completed this in July, just two weeks after my last dose of chemotherapy. I ran the whole race without stopping and did it in thirty-four minutes. I was so proud of myself; this gave me a much-needed boost.

In August, just six months after my fortieth birthday, I organized a huge Bollywood-themed bash with costumes and music. I even decorated the garden in a Bollywood style. It was just the best night ever and so nice to be able to have fun with friends and family again. We then had a big family holiday to Cyprus in October after another 'clear' scan. We made sure the next Christmas was fabulous, to make up for the previous year. I couldn't believe the difference a year made. Yes, I was still tired, yes, scarred for life, but here I was alive, happy and with hope for the future.

Now yet another year has passed and we have a family holiday booked at Easter. I thankfully had another 'clear' scan in January and my next one is due in May.

Keeping up with fitness, and feeling spurred on to help others, I have even signed up to do a triathlon. So now I'm regularly running, swimming and cycling.

James and I are also riding tandem from London to Brighton soon to raise more money and awareness for a pancreatic cancer charity.

It hasn't been easy; in fact, at times I felt like giving up. I've had no one really to talk to who can fully appreciate how awful this insidious disease is. Unfortunately, only three percent of people with pancreatic cancer live five years or more. Despite being fully aware of this, I always smile and have never given up; I push myself constantly.

I really believe a positive attitude can help beat cancer.

MIRACLES DO HAPPEN

MEMBERSHIP: # 15

I was watching television with my husband one evening, when I idly rubbed the left side of my face. I felt a small lump about the size of a grape. I thought it was odd but assumed I had maybe bumped into something unknowingly. The lump was at the entrance to my ear. After a few days, it still hadn't gone, so I made an appointment to see my doctor. He was brilliant and referred me to an Ear, Nose and Throat (ENT) consultant straight away. An appointment came through for the end of October.

One morning at the beginning of October, I again visited my doctor. This time I had a rather uncomfortable pain in my groin area, which ran down my leg. However, I wasn't able to pinpoint exactly where the pain was coming from. The doctor thought it was just some kind of groin strain and it would ease over time by itself. But within just a few hours I was in absolute agony. The pain had now become localized on my right side. I went back to my doctor who wasted no time in booking me into the Gynaecology Department at the local hospital as an emergency case. He suspected it might be an ovarian cyst. I underwent several examinations including a scan and everything was still suggesting his first diagnosis was correct. So they decided to operate to remove the cyst. I was told I would have a procedure called a laparoscopy, which would mean being under anaesthetic for about thirty minutes, depending on what they found.

The advantage of a laparoscopy is that it is a relatively non-invasive procedure. Typically, a small incision is made just below the navel and a cannula or trocar is inserted into the incision to accommodate the insertion of the laparoscope. Other incisions may be made in the abdomen to allow the insertion of additional laparoscopic instruments. However, if they found something, they'd have to open me right up. If this happened, then obviously the operation would take much longer.

When I came round from the anaesthetic, the first thing I did was check the time. It was nearly three hours since I'd been taken down to theatre. I instantly started panicking, wondering what they'd done and if I'd had a hysterectomy.

When the consultant visited me, she explained that when they did the laparoscopy everything was bulging towards the camera. Yet curiously, when they opened me up to remove what they were sure was a large cyst, there was nothing there. I'd been through all this for nothing and felt so frustrated and angry. I was in hospital for a total of ten days as I managed to pick up an infection, too – great!

It was now the end of October and I had my next appointment with the ENT consultant. He gave me a very thorough examination, sticking things up my nose, down my throat and in my ears. He also did a needle aspiration on the lump and said he'd decide what to do after the results came back from the laboratories. I received a letter that said the sample had shown 'rather odd cells' and that I'd been booked into hospital again in February, this time to have the lump removed from the side of my face.

Two weeks before the operation was due, the lump disappeared. When I went to see the consultant, he said, 'Oh, well, looks like you've saved yourself an operation.'

He decided to just keep an eye on me and a follow-up appointment was made, for six months' time.

My life continued as normal until about two weeks before the follow-up appointment, when yet again I felt a lump. This time, it was just to the left of my neck. With lumps also coming and going in my groin area and neck, I started to do a bit of reading myself; everything I found on the internet pointed towards my having a lymphoma-type cancer. Lymphoma meant cancer of the lymphatic system of which there are two main types. They are called Hodgkin Lymphoma or Non-Hodgkin Lymphoma (NHL).

I went to my appointment and the hospital registrar saw me. He felt the lump in my neck and put it down to swollen glands and told me to come back in three months' time. The next appointment soon came round and the lump was still there. Luckily, I saw the same registrar and again he said it was just a swollen gland. Well, this time I wasn't so sure, so asked him about lymphoma cancer and if he'd ruled it out.

He chuckled a bit and said, 'You're no more likely to have lymphoma than myself or the nurse here. But clearly you're worried so would you like me to see you again in January?'

'Yes please,' I replied instantly.

Finally, in January, it was decided that a biopsy of the swelling was needed and an operation was booked. I visited the hospital for the results in March. I remember the date well as it was my dad's fiftieth birthday. The news was not good – as I had suspected I was diagnosed with lymphoma. I had Non-Hodgkin, large B-cell, to be precise. I was told at the time that this was the more aggressive type but the one that was easier to cure. I was being referred to the Haematology Department for my treatment, but it would be a long haul and I would get extremely tired and sick. They didn't exactly make it sound like something enjoyable or fun.

Cancer is one of those things that you always believe won't happen to you. Other people get cancer, not you. When I was told I had cancer, my immediate thought was: 'Oh my God, I'm going to die.' This was followed by despair, anger, and questions like: 'Why me?' I don't smoke, I don't drink to excess and I eat fairly healthily.

I went to meet the consultant who was going to be looking after me. She explained all about the disease and how we were going to fight it. She was very positive and encouraging, which helped me enormously. The next thing they needed to do was stage me and give me the dreaded bone marrow test.

I underwent six courses of CHOP chemotherapy and was fortunate that the only side effect I noticed was hair loss. This was followed by two weeks of radiotherapy. During the course of my treatment, I also had a stem cell harvest, just as a precaution against future complications.

After a CT scan, I was told the amazing news that I was in remission. I'd done it – the relief was indescribable. I couldn't think of anything better to do than celebrate.

Sadly, one casualty of my illness was my marriage – life-changing experiences such as cancer can either make or break a couple; unfortunately, it broke us. Different people cope in different ways. However, on a positive note, I soon met Mark and we moved in together, choosing his home town as our base.

I was very nervous about handing my follow-up care to doctors that I didn't know, or them me.

My current consultant recommended a hospital and put me in touch with the appropriate person.

All continued well with life and my health until February, some five years later. We were staying in Devon for the weekend when I noticed an uncomfortable swelling under my arm. I felt sick to the pit of my stomach, and my heart sank; I instinctively knew what the problem would be. As soon as we got home from Devon, I rang the hospital. They told me to come and see them straight away.

The consultant could definitely feel something, but until a biopsy was taken he was obviously unable to say what. We had a week's holiday planned in Majorca and the operation date typically came through for that week. When I rang and explained the situation, it transpired the next available date was a further six weeks later. We couldn't take the risk of waiting that long, so arranged a private operation for the week after our holiday. Majorca was fantastic; we went with some very good friends and it was just what I needed – anything to take my mind off my situation. On the flight home, I had terrible earache following the landing and could still feel a small lump in that area. I'd hoped like last time the lump might have magically disappeared.

The operation itself went well but I developed an infection and ended up being off work for over two weeks. When we went to get the results, the news wasn't good. The cancer had returned, but with a twist. This time it was Follicular Non-Hodgkin Lymphoma. I mentioned the lump by my ear and was told it felt like bone and was probably nothing to worry about. After the staging, it was decided that the best plan of action was a course of chlorambucil chemotherapy taken orally. No hair loss, no sickness, in fact virtually no side effects at all – perfect. Maybe it wasn't so bad, I thought. I had to go for regular checks while taking the drug. Each time, I mentioned the lump by my ear, as it was getting bigger. After the fifth check-up, one of the registrars decided that something needed to be done. She conversed with my consultant and a third biopsy was planned.

The lump was in my right parotid gland. The facial nerve runs right through it, so there was a danger of facial palsy following the operation. The last thing I needed was facial muscle weakness or even eye closure. Thankfully, I escaped this and everything was fine.

Yes, it was Follicular Lymphoma. It was decided that a blast of radiotherapy to the area would be a good idea. Because it was to be aimed at my face, it would go across my eyes. This could possibly cause me to develop cataracts in around three or so years' time. I felt I could handle that, as I knew they are able to remove these easily enough nowadays. All the planning was done and I had a mask made. This was about 7 cm by 6 cm in size and covered part of my face, something that was needed for the radiotherapy.

On the day of the first dose of radiation, the doctor in charge pulled me aside and said she was not happy about giving me such a large dose and wanted my consultant to review his decision. He took one look at me and decided the best course of action would now be a stronger form of chemotherapy, called FMD. I had the first dose just before Christmas. It worked, thankfully; the lump virtually disappeared with just one treatment.

Obviously, I had to finish the course to gain the most benefit, but we were all really excited.

We had a holiday booked for the Christmas and now maybe I could relax and enjoy it. The holiday was wonderful and, to my delight, Mark proposed. We came home to family that were thrilled by our news. We hadn't set a date but were both thinking between three to five years' time – once things had settled down more with both work and life in general. I have to admit that there was a part of me that thought I may not be here in three years' time, but I tried desperately to keep really positive and kept these feelings to myself.

The chemotherapy was at intervals of four weeks, and by the time the next dose was due the lump had returned. We plodded on with the treatment and I had all four doses before it became obvious it wasn't working; yet another setback. My consultant was a little baffled and wanted to take another biopsy. My scans had shown the area in my abdomen appeared to be relatively stable.

The results of the biopsy were confirmed – my large B-cell had returned, so I was given a more aggressive chemotherapy. Whether it was there all the time or the cancer had developed since last time wasn't clear.

Rituximab had been approved by NICE in November; we were now in June of the following year. I would be having five doses of RCHOP. This was the most I could have as I'd already had six doses of a chemotherapy called CHOP a few years ago. Following that, they recommended I have a stem cell transplant. This was planned for the September. I don't tend to make things easy for myself.

During August, I was online casually looking at properties in Devon, as Mark and I were thinking of moving back to the area. Ideally, we wanted it to coincide with my eldest starting high school. I came across a property that was absolutely perfect. Mark wanted somewhere that was going to earn us a living; we needed a large house because of the six children we had between us. More importantly, it had to fit our budget. This property met our criteria and more. I printed off the details and showed them to Mark saying that it was the kind of place we needed. Mark agreed it was perfect, and thought we might not find anything as suitable again. We could always rent it out until we were ready to move in. Anyway, one thing led to another and we decided that if the place was so right for us why not move now, so we made an offer. It was accepted around the beginning of September.

Because I was so far down the line with my treatment, I thought it would be sensible to carry on having the transplant done in the North, at my current hospital. So there I was sorting out new schools and arranging a house move all before I went into hospital for the transplant. Our completion date for the house was set for the beginning of October, which meant the house contents would move, followed by me a couple of days later. As the transplant date I had been given was for the Monday, I thought I had a whole weekend to sort things out. However, I received a phone call asking if I could go in earlier as a bed might not be available on the Monday. I didn't have any choice really, so was admitted to hospital on Friday, 17 September.

My mum was fantastic and told me not to worry as she'd sort out all the moving arrangements for me.

My treatment started on the Sunday night and initially I didn't feel too bad; well, I hadn't been sick. I started to go downhill after about ten days. I had put on a lot of weight because of all the previous treatment in the run-up to the transplant. In addition, my body started to retain a lot of fluid. I also felt breathless and didn't want to speak to people on the phone because it was such an effort. I'd gone off my food and felt very low. I wanted to be with someone all the time and wanted someone to stay with me overnight. Mark was fantastic, especially as when we first met he told me he 'didn't do hospitals'. He stayed every night in my room on a put-up bed. In the mornings, he would race home to wash. He wasn't allowed to use my bathroom because I was toxic and could contaminate him, and I risked picking up an infection. Mark would try to fit in a day's work and be back at the hospital for seven each evening.

After about two weeks, I had what I describe as a funny turn. I was not really aware of my surroundings all morning and my breathing had rapidly deteriorated. A crash team soon arrived and I was given oxygen; there was an air of panic in my room. The crash team managed to stabilize me but wanted me to be admitted to the Intensive Care Unit (ICU). However, because my resistance to infection was at its lowest point, they couldn't take the chance of taking me out of isolation. After a while, I had an x-ray, ECGs, scans and a heart echo test. They concluded my heart had been damaged by the chemotherapy and some of the tablets were affecting my kidneys so they weren't functioning correctly. This explained why I had retained so much fluid. They didn't seem overly concerned and told me that, as I recovered, got fitter and started moving around, the fluid would eventually disperse. Over time, my blood counts gradually improved, and on 9 October I was discharged with a large bag of pills to take.

I still had what the doctors called oedema, which was an excess retention of fluid. Added to this, I still was not very mobile. I needed a wheelchair to leave the hospital; Mark managed to get me into the car. We drove straight to our new home in Devon. Mum and Dad and all our children were there to greet me, so it was a very emotional homecoming.

I still wasn't well and Mum was really worried; I had no interest in anything. I was not eating properly and it was an enormous effort just to get upstairs to bed; breathing was still one of my big problems, too.

It was my birthday on 11 October and I didn't even open my presents, I just felt so ill. Because the doctors had said I'd get better, I plodded on thinking it was just a matter of time. By this point, I now weighed a massive eighteen stone. I had put on over two stone while in hospital. I'd been home for just five days, and was busy trying to help get the house sorted, when I had my first follow-up appointment. Mum had driven me there that afternoon and, while I was waiting to see the consultant, I rapidly deteriorated. I was taken to a side room in the Haematology Ward and the duty doctor explained to Mum that it was not looking good. Mark was away at the time. By the time he arrived at the hospital, doctors wanted to get me into ICU; however, there was only one bed available and two patients, including me, needing it. The staff nurse on the ward tried her best to slow down my breathing. She eventually thought I was going to have heart failure and called the crash team.

The next thing I remember is being raced through the hospital with what felt like a black bag over my face.

Some three weeks later, I was still in ICU. I was on a ventilator and had been since my last memory of my face being covered. Apparently, the doctors weren't holding out much hope for me in the first few days. At one point, they even talked about turning off the life-support machine. Slowly, I improved but I contracted a horrendous infection in my central lines and other tubes; these were soon taken out.

Mark and Mum were still being prepared for the possibility that I might not survive. I spent a total of four weeks in ICU and a further two weeks on the Cardiac Ward. The conclusion was I'd had heart failure due to the chemotherapy. My heart was beating way too fast and not sufficient for my lungs, which had filled with fluid. The ventilator basically stopped me from drowning. While I was in intensive care, the doctors slowly managed to get most of the fluid out of my system. I lost a total of four stone in four weeks; now that's what I call a diet.

When the sedation was lifted, I realized I was unable to move; I couldn't even roll over in bed or dress myself. On the ward, I had to learn this all over again, like a baby learning to walk, before I could be discharged. I was desperate to go home as by this time I was actually feeling better than I had done for months. Being an extremely determined person, just four days after being admitted on the ward, I took my first couple of steps with a walking frame. After that, there was no stopping me; before they knew it, I was walking to the end of the corridor and back.

I was finally discharged just before Christmas, but still needed the walking frame.

Mark moved the bed into the lounge so I didn't need to worry about climbing the stairs.

We had most of the family stay with us over the Christmas period. I set myself the goal of conquering the stairs by then, which I somehow achieved.

All the doctors have been amazed at my recovery; they call me 'miracle lady'. I'm still a bit weak but am walking unaided, can do most things for myself and am leading a fairly normal life. I have no breathing difficulties now and, even better, it seems the cancer is still nowhere to be seen, which my last scans confirmed. I have to take rather a lot of tablets but I can cope with that.

Yet again, good things have come from me being ill, as I believe they always do. Mark and I got married last summer; life is too short to wait any longer. I have made a wonderful new friend via the Lymphoma Association website. I started logging onto their site during my treatment. I needed information and was desperate to talk to people who knew what

I was going through. It's not a busy website and sometimes it's weeks before there's anyone else online, too. One night a woman appeared online and we got on really well. Apart from the obvious subject of lymphoma, we found we had so many other things in common. She also lives quite close so we now often meet up and have a good gossip. She was very supportive throughout my treatment and we met for real in ICU, so she saw me at my worst.

Where we are living is so idyllic and I love our house. We almost have our own little valley; we can't see any other properties and no one can see us.

The children are going to the same primary school that I went to and have settled in well. We live just fifteen minutes from all my immediate family.

Someone somewhere has really been looking out for me; I feel very humbled by that knowledge. The support I received from family, friends and complete strangers was amazing. I feel very privileged to have received that, and despite being ill I am a very lucky lady. I now want to try to help others, to repay those who helped me when I was ill.

FLOWERS, CAKES AND COTTON BUDS

MEMBERSHIP: # 1

V isitors are banned from taking flowers into our hospitals. We're told it reduces the chances of patients suffering a slow and painful death, should they contract the highly contagious 'wilting petal' disease. The ban was enforced despite the Department of Health issuing a statement saying, 'There's no evidence of flower water causing an infection.' What a surprise – I often thought people confused a vase containing flowers with a water jug...

Now, some hospitals have banned homemade cakes because of health and safety concerns. Officials claim sponge cakes contravene guidelines, blaming the ban on strict rules over packaging and labelling.

What the Department of Health and Safety has failed to

notice, due to its obsession with creating legislation on our every activity, is that it is breeding a new highly contagious disease. It's far more dangerous than any 'wilting petal' disease. It's called moron's disease. I'm not talking about the city in Argentina; I'm talking about people of subnormal intelligence. That's politically correct speak for idiot, thick or stupid.

Now, when we purchase a hot drink, we need to be told we could burn ourselves. When crossing a road, we have to be told which way to look. The funniest warning I read was in a car handbook, which stated, 'For safety reasons, carry out engine adjustments while the vehicle is stationary.'

The compulsive preoccupation with making us all healthier and safer is actually creating an unhealthy and unsafe nation of idiots, who are becoming unable to think for themselves.

Over 7,000 people with moron's disease attended Accident & Emergency last year to have cotton buds removed from their ears. That's more than the number of people who had accidents with razor blades. The official explanation is razor blades have a warning on the packet, cotton buds don't.

Ready meals have instructions on both opening and cooking the contents, because six out of ten people have stabbed themselves when trying to open a ready meal with a knife; and that's with instructions.

I was in a meeting this week with the marketing team of 'Above and Beyond', a charity that raises and manages funds for all nine hospitals in the University Hospitals Bristol NHS Foundation Trust. I jokingly suggested they put a leaflet under the pillow of all the patients, a little like the flyers we get stuffed under our windscreen wipers in car parks. I was told they'd need to be laminated, because of, you've guessed it, 'Health and Safety'.

However, it's OK for an uninvited stranger to stuff a leaflet through my letter box, advertising a 'No win no fee' service, should I be the victim of medical negligence. Yet, if they slip on my garden path, they're entitled to claim damages from me.

Relax, before you get stressed because you weren't warned this column could increase your blood pressure. I have a solution – I have a vaccine for the 2.7 million people who visit A & E with moron's disease each year. It's called common sense.

Finally, I'd like to congratulate you on your bravery in reading this newspaper today.

To think, without any words of caution you risked paper cuts, ink coming off on your hands and me waffling on about morons.

BETTER YOU THAN ME

MEMBERSHIP: # 16

My illness started when I was just ten years old. I was staying over at a friend's house one weekend. I woke up on the Sunday morning being sick and I couldn't stop; it was really embarrassing. I went home assuming I'd picked up a bug and felt well enough for school by Monday.

As the weeks drifted on, I continued being sick, which by then had become almost a daily event. Mum eventually took me to the doctor's, but they were unable to find anything wrong. Mum kept wondering if I was being bullied at school, which wasn't the case. I carried on going to school as normal but was still being sick on a regular basis. To add to this, I started getting severe headaches, so Mum kept taking me back to the doctor's. Eventually, I was told I was having 'migraines of the stomach'.

My doctor prescribed some tablets; however, my symptoms continued and actually got worse. Then I began to experience pains in my lower back and struggled to keep my balance. I wasn't even able to walk in a straight line without stumbling all over the place. It must have looked like I was drunk, except I wasn't even old enough to drink alcohol!

Despite my growing list of problems, nobody believed I was genuinely unwell. My symptoms continued and I got progressively worse. The constant sickness meant I was unable to keep any food down, which in turn meant I lost a lot of weight. Soon after this my speech became slurred and I was now looking and sounding like a drunk. At the time I guessed this must be what a hangover felt like: now, sadly, I've first-hand knowledge!

Most mornings, I'd visit my doctor, yet they were still unable to diagnose what was causing my now numerous problems. Still they insisted I was simply having these 'migraines of the stomach'. My symptoms and regular doctors' appointments continued for several more months. I'd see the doctor before school then spend the rest of the day acting like the local drunk; it felt like I had the worst hangover in the world.

Eventually, after numerous appointments, I was referred to the hospital. By this point, I was really ill. I was constantly being sick, slurring my speech and unable to walk properly. My 'migraines' had become so bad I could barely lift my head off a cushion, which I used to keep the light out of my eyes. Just when I thought I couldn't feel any worse, yet another symptom appeared: one of my eyes started to turn in. I was forced to sit at the front of the classroom in order to see. I even needed to cover my bad eye when watching television as it hurt so much. The combination of all these symptoms was really starting to affect my life now.

Coincidently, the night before my hospital appointment, I watched a television programme about a young girl, who was around my age. She'd been having similar symptoms to me and was diagnosed with a brain tumour. This really frightened me. I remember asking Mum if this could be causing all my problems. She dismissed the idea instantly, explaining I'd not been experiencing projectile vomiting like the young girl had. I was unable to watch the rest of the programme, my imagination getting the better of me. I went upstairs to bed and tried to forget about my hospital appointment the next morning.

Mum and I arrived at the hospital early and, after a short wait, a nurse performed various tests. Then we had an agonizing wait to see the consultant. The consultant tested my reflexes and checked my eyes. He then startled me by saying he needed a second opinion. This naturally frightened me; my mind went back to the girl I'd watched on television the night before. Eventually, the second consultant arrived and looked into my eyes. I was then asked if I'd wait outside while they discussed my symptoms in more detail.

After more waiting around, they explained it would help them with my diagnosis if I had an MRI scan. This would be done at a different hospital. I felt fine about having the scan, until I saw the size of the massive machine. A nurse wanted me to lie on a moving couch, which would slide inside a tunnel; I was really terrified by now. After discussing it in detail with the nurse, she convinced me I'd be fine and able to cope with any possible claustrophobic feeling, and she was right.

Once the scan was over, the consultant called me into his

small office. I had both Mum and my stepdad with me for support. Before I'd even had time to take in my surroundings, the consultant announced, 'I'm sorry, Abbie, but it looks like you have a brain tumour.'

I can still picture him telling me as if it was today. Initially, I was relieved; at last they'd found out what was causing all my problems. I couldn't think properly as thoughts about dying raced around my head. I had no idea if they could cure me or get the lump out and I'd never felt my heart beat so fast. The consultant explained an ambulance was on its way, as I needed an operation.

This was to be done at another hospital that specialized in neurosurgery, and the operation was scheduled for the following morning.

That night, Mum went home as there was nothing more she could do. It was an awful feeling being alone in hospital, knowing I had an operation the next day. As you can imagine, I didn't sleep much. I sat around watching videos and chatting with the nurses.

Mum and my stepdad arrived early the next morning and the three of us talked with the surgeon. Mum signed some authorization forms and then soon enough I was being wheeled down to theatre. Almost twelve hours later, I woke up in the High Dependency Unit (HDU). I'm told the first thing I asked Mum was 'What's the time?' Then I instantly fell back to sleep before she had time to answer. It's strange the things we say when coming round from an operation. I was obviously unaware of what I was saying and I don't remember too much about my stay on the HDU, as I'd been kept heavily sedated.

After a few days, I was moved to the Intensive Care Unit (ICU) where I was constantly monitored and connected to a self-dispensing morphine machine, to help me cope with the pain. The nurses regularly moved me so I didn't get bed sores and regularly changed my dressings. Once I was well enough, I was moved to a normal ward. Here I started my recovery properly. Soon I was able to eat again but the hospital food wasn't that great. Luckily, my dear mum would bring food from the hospital café, which was much better. I then started to put weight on and gain enough strength to enable me to walk again. My stay in hospital seemed to last forever, despite having lots of people visit me each day.

I was finally discharged from hospital, having spent ten very long days there.

After leaving hospital, my progress continued and I began eating normal-size portions again. I was given steroids to take and strangely noticed I had a craving for bacon sandwiches and hot chocolate.

A few weeks later, I started back at school. Unfortunately, it hadn't been possible to remove all of the cancerous cells during my operation, so I was told I'd need a course of radiotherapy next. A metal mask was made, to make sure I stayed perfectly still and didn't move while having the radiotherapy treatment. First, a mould of my face was made from wet plaster. This was placed over my face until it had dried. It wasn't a pleasant experience and I remember crying the moment I got out of the hospital that day. When I next saw the mask, I noticed how the eyes, nose and mouth had all been cleverly cut out of the mould ready for me to wear.

My radiotherapy treatment lasted a total of six weeks. I used to have it in the mornings before school. It was actually OK having the radiotherapy and not as scary as I'd imagined. However, it wasn't nice being pinned down on a hard surface, but I knew the treatment would eliminate any chance of the cancer coming back and growing again.

Once my treatment was over, I started having check-ups every week, seeing lots of different doctors and always worried what they'd find each time.

The operation had appeared to cause a few problems with my growth. I'd stopped getting taller and was put on a growth hormone, which had to be injected; ouch! Eventually, I learnt to do this myself, which made life easier.

Unfortunately, I also suffered from depression so saw a psychologist, who suggested I change school. I was moved to a hospital school with only six people in my class. This helped me with my learning but I still got depressed and kept crying at the most inappropriate of things. I guess I had been through a lot at such a young age.

The first six years of remission were quite hectic, as I learnt to cope with the side effects and tried to get my life back to normal.

Thirteen years on, I'm now twenty-three and feeling the best I have ever felt. I still get down occasionally but I'm so thankful just to be here. I am currently training to be a paramedic and am really looking forward to a career helping people.

I now live each day as if it's my last; I appreciate how lucky I am to be alive and no longer take life for granted. If you're reading this having been diagnosed with cancer, trust me, it's worth the fight. Life will be so much more enjoyable and never again will you feel daunted or think you're unable to achieve your goals or dreams!

I must thank my surgeon and doctors for saving my life and thank all my family for helping me; especially my mum.

MOTHER OF ALL SURGERIES

MEMBERSHIP: # 17

It all started quite dramatically for me two years ago in May. It was a normal Saturday morning and I was out with my family shopping. Around 9:30 A.M., having only just arrived at the shops, I started to feel unwell. I was experiencing pains in my tummy and felt hot and really quite uncomfortable. We cut our shopping trip short and quickly made our way back home. By the time we arrived, I was in quite a lot of pain, feeling even hotter and very light-headed. For the next forty-odd minutes, I was literally rolling around on the bedroom floor, as the pain increased. Eventually, I asked Tracey, my wife, to call an ambulance, as I simply couldn't handle the sheer agony any more.

The ambulance crew soon arrived and suggested they take me to the local Accident & Emergency Department. My brother also came over to look after our daughters, Jessica and Chloe. I was soon loaded into the ambulance, and Tracey and my parents followed behind in their car. On the way to the hospital, the ambulance crew gave me something for the pain. I was now shaking uncontrollably and felt absolutely awful. On arrival, I was given some morphine and the doctors examined me. Various tests were carried out and they slowly got my pain under control.

About an hour and a half later, a doctor explained that they were unsure what had caused my problems. They felt as the pain had subsided it would be safe for me to go back home. I'd fully expected they'd want to keep me in for the night. Anyway, I got dressed and made my way back out to the car.

I was still feeling very fragile and tender, making walking difficult. In the car park, I spotted the ambulance crew who'd helped me; they were surprised that I was going home so soon.

For the rest of the weekend, I was in a lot of discomfort, feeling feverish and off my food; most unlike me.

It soon became obvious on Monday morning that I'd be unable to go to work. I couldn't even get my trousers on as I was still in so much pain. I needed to see my local doctor as clearly I was unwell, it was obvious now I had more than just food poisoning.

I was lucky enough to get an emergency appointment and saw the doctor early. I explained to her what had happened over the weekend and she felt I needed to go back to the hospital. To her, it was clear I was unwell and my symptoms concerned her. I was given a letter and she explained I should go to the Surgical Admissions Ward, which I found worrying.

When I was admitted to the ward, both Tracey and Mum were with me. A doctor examined me and requested more tests and for an x-ray to be taken. I was also given a drip as I was dehydrated due to being unable to eat or drink much. The doctor came back later with three medical students, who all took it in turn to examine me. The doctor asked the students to explain what they were doing and looking for. When the doctor asked one of the students what she thought the problem was, she said she thought I had peritonitis.

'Spot on,' the doctor replied. 'What makes you think that?'

'Rebound tests show a reaction, he's hot, dehydrated and has abdominal pain.'

'Good, but there is one thing you have missed: look at his skin colour. He's yellow, almost jaundice-like, and the whites of his eyes are yellow, too. Mr Mason, you need an operation quite quickly to remove your appendix; we'll aim to have you in theatre by midnight tonight,' the doctor said, while the students gazed at me in silence.

I could hear the blood rushing around my head and my heart beating really fast now as the shock of his news sank in.

The reality was that I didn't get operated on until the Tuesday morning, at around 9:30 A.M. This was nearly four days after my appendix had perforated. I was really unwell during the night, so it was decided that I should have some intravenous antibiotics.

The surgery went well but wasn't straightforward. While I was still in the recovery ward, a doctor came to see me. He said the laparoscopy had taken around an hour and a half longer than normal. The appendix had stuck to both my ileum and caecum, which had to be cut away. Apart from that, the operation had been a success. Later, I was moved to a general ward for recovery, where I spent the next week on high-dose antibiotics and sporting a stomach drain. I was then finally discharged.

The events of the last week had been a shock and totally unexpected. The knowledge that I was on the mend and the operation was behind me aided my recovery. Three weeks after the operation, I returned to work and started to get back to normal. I began to exercise and was eager to put the whole horrible appendix experience behind me.

Slowly, I felt unwell again, but just assumed I'd maybe been pushing myself a little too hard.

To my surprise, I received a letter asking me to attend an out-patient appointment at the colorectal unit at the hospital. The same day, I received a phone call asking that I also have a CT scan. I assumed this was simply a routine procedure that everyone had and was impressed with the aftercare service the NHS offered.

As it was a late afternoon, I attended the out-patient appointment on my own, on my way home from work. It was a perfect hot July day and the waiting room was full. Typically, all the appointments were running late. I sat quietly reading old magazines and people watching until my name was called. I casually made my way to the appointment office and was introduced to the specialist colorectal nurse and the consultant. Their mood was a little sombre but I didn't think too much about it. After some polite chat about the weather, they explained that my appendix had been sent to the lab for a biopsy. This was routine procedure after an operation, but they'd found a problem. My heart started beating a little faster as beads of sweat began forming on my face. The lab found that I had a mucinous cystadenoma with associated low-grade mucinous adenocarcinoma. I had no idea what that meant but the doctors sounded confident.

I remember hearing the word cancer being mentioned. Stupidly, I just couldn't think straight as I tried to comprehend everything they were telling me. I also remembered being told that I'd need to have a CT scan before they'd know more. I told them I already had an appointment for this. The most shocking news was they felt I'd need a colonoscopy and very likely another operation called a right hemicolectomy. Now I was very confused and sweat was pouring down my face. He said that a hemicolectomy was an operation on my colon, which they would do by making an incision via my abdomen. The CT scan, along with the colonoscopy, would give doctors more of an idea of my problem, enabling them to put a care plan together. I was briefly examined and they were happy with the way I was recovering from the appendectomy. I walked back to the car in a state of shock. I was thinking I'd just been told I had cancer. I was in such shock I didn't really listen or understand exactly everything they'd said.

As I drove home, typically the roads were congested. It was very hot and I was fighting back the tears. My biggest concern now was how I was going to tell Tracey. I arrived home to find her and the girls enjoying the weather in the garden. Tracey looked stunning sunning herself and the girls were happily playing together. I discreetly asked Tracey to come inside as I wanted to talk.

'Come inside?' she queried. Instantly, she guessed something was wrong.

We went into the front room and I burst out crying before we'd even sat down. I explained what had happened at the hospital. Tracey kept asking questions I couldn't answer as I hadn't really absorbed everything I was told. She was obviously upset and I felt so bad for making her cry. The girls kept coming inside as they could sense there was a problem but eventually we managed to get them to go back outside and play.

I called my parents and brother and asked if they'd come round. That evening, I told them my news and the three of them were devastated. Both Tracey and I were now feeling very down and depressed. The shock and mental stress of the appendectomy was only just subsiding and suddenly I was told I had cancer. I don't mind admitting the news had really stunned me. I felt sick to the pit of my stomach. So many things ran through my mind. The obvious first questions I had were 'Why me?' and 'Am I going to die?' I'd known people who had suffered from cancer, fought hard, but still died. I didn't want to be like them.

The day of my CT scan appointment soon arrived. I sat in the waiting room; thankfully, only a couple of other people were there. A lady sitting opposite me was clearly undergoing chemotherapy. Her skin was grey; she looked very thin and wore a headscarf. I wondered if that would be me soon, but without the headscarf, obviously.

A week or so later, another appointment letter arrived; this time, I had to see a consultant and specialist nurse. The hospital called and suggested Tracey accompany me. This was mainly to make sure we came away from the meeting fully understanding everything that had been discussed.

We arrived at the hospital and made our way to the Colorectal Ward. The wait to be seen felt like years, not minutes. We walked through the consultant's office and into a lounge, well, a very comfy little room anyway. My heart sank. I instantly knew what this all meant. The consultant did most of the talking. He explained that the CT scan had shown a mucinous-like jelly, coating my organs in the abdominal cavity. He said it was a very rare type of cancer, known as Pseudomyxoma Peritonei (PMP). It only affects one in every million people and can't be treated by conventional chemotherapy. Instead, the usual treatment for PMP is a huge operation known as the 'Sugarbaker Technique'. Due to the seriousness of the operation and the expertise required, it would have to be performed at a specialist centre in Basingstoke. This I later found out was one of only two hospitals in the country that could do the operation at the time. The Christie Hospital in Manchester was the other.

Tracey was by now crying and I was also very close to tears myself. This was bad. 'So what are my chances?' I asked.

'You're a prime candidate for the operation – fit, young and well – but people can die from this condition. The other thing we must stress is that it is a very slow-growing cancer.'

Everything else he said became blurred again. However, we were given a very useful information booklet about the condition and contact details of the specialist nurse in Basingstoke, who would now be looking after me. Yet another appointment was made, this time to meet the team in Basingstoke. Still trying to take in the news, we composed ourselves and left the hospital. This was easily the lowest we'd ever felt. We got outside and Tracey broke down. I held her tight and we cried together. We felt like our whole world had just been shattered.

After several weeks of waiting, I finally attended my first appointment at Basingstoke in August. The consultant asked me to explain the sequence of events leading up to my appendix perforating. He examined me and discussed in detail the various aspects of PMP, while looking at my CT images. He explained that PMP was very slow growing. I had evidence of it around my liver, stomach, spleen and in my pelvis. The right side of my abdomen was pretty clear as this had probably been cleared out during the appendectomy. He advised that the small amount of fluid found had probably been in my abdomen for around five to ten years. He said the operation was known among PMP sufferers as the Mother of All Surgeries (MOAS). I let out a nervous laugh, while the blood drained from Tracey's face. He felt I'd probably need a number of procedures, including: a midline laparotomy with excision of the umbilicus, a stripping of my diaphragm, a diathermy liver capsulectomy, a cholecystectomy, a greater and lesser omentectomy, and either a diathermy capsulectomy of the spleen or spleenectomy. Also I'd need a right hemicolectomy or possible excision of the appendix stump and finally a possible anterior resection. It all sounded double Dutch to me. I might as well have been listening to one of those 'Teach Yourself' language CDs.

If all the disease was successfully removed, it was thought an hour of intra-operative chemotherapy and possibly some post-operative chemotherapy would be all that was needed. It was decided a second CT scan should be done in October, as there is often a lot of fluid left in the abdomen after the initial appendectomy and there was a slim chance my body could reabsorb this fluid. If the fluid remained or grew, however, I would need to go ahead with the operation.

This meeting had been far more upbeat and positive. The

team appeared confident that something could be done, but obviously they could give no guarantees. The statistics showed two out of three people who had this operation would remain disease free at three years. The odds didn't seem totally stacked against me after all. Both Tracey and I felt much better and a little happier than we had for a long time.

I had the second CT scan and, unfortunately, the fluid had not been reabsorbed, so the inevitable (MOAS) operation was definitely on. It wasn't something they'd rush to do, which gave me time to prepare.

'The letter' arrived in December – some Christmas card that was. I was to be admitted on 31 January and my operation would go ahead on 2 February. Despite this news, we did have a great Christmas. We made an extra effort to ensure we had fun. We organized games and a Christmas quiz to liven up the whole day, which the girls really enjoyed. We spent New Year's Eve with a group of friends at our local rugby club. When midnight arrived, we had a few tearful moments before we got on with the task of enjoying ourselves.

Throughout January, I kept busy at work, preparing for the six months I'd be out of action. All the time I was fully aware that the MOAS was looming ever closer, which I obviously couldn't stop thinking about. On my last day at work at the end of January, my colleagues gave me a great send-off. I was very emotional, yet it was also a brilliant and memorable day.

I now only had one week until the operation and started to get ready. I sorted out my bags and packed them with plenty of DVDs, books and magazines to keep me occupied. The hardest thing I did by far was to write letters to Tracey and my two daughters, Jessica and Chloe. Just in case things didn't go my way and I didn't return home. It was a worrying time. I spent a whole afternoon in the bedroom in tears, doing my best to put my feelings into words. This was an awful and very difficult experience. Unable to sleep at night, I resorted to using some chemical help prescribed by the doctor. I didn't want to go into an operation already exhausted through lack of sleep. It was important that I was well rested.

Eventually, the day I had been dreading arrived. I was all packed and ready to go. My parents arrived to collect us. We wanted to get on the road early to avoid the rush-hour traffic. It also meant we got our goodbyes to the family out of the way quickly and didn't have time to think about things too much. I held my girls tight and again couldn't help crying. This I prayed wouldn't be the last time I held them. I tore myself away and we got into the car and were soon on our way.

Tracey and Mum checked into the on-site accommodation, as they were going to stay with me while I was hospitalized. I headed towards Ward C2, the specialist Pseudomyxoma Peritonei Unit. Here I was shown to my private room with en suite. Throughout the day, various people came to speak with me and lots of tests were performed. In addition, I had to sign the consent forms and was now only allowed a diet of clear fluids.

The following day, I was visited by the surgical team, anaesthetist, stoma nurse, physiotherapist and many other staff. There were five separate consultants on the team, as well as the specialist nurses. That evening, we were given a tour of the Intensive Care Unit (ICU) so we could see where it was and get used to the environment where I'd wake following the operation. Each bed was attended by one member of staff and the atmosphere was surprisingly relaxed, which was reassuring.

On 2 February, the nurses woke me early, allowing me time to get up and have a shower. I surprised myself by how relaxed I was. I think by now I knew I was prepared as much physically and mentally as I would ever be. I just wanted the operation all over with. Tracey and Mum arrived to see me off. I was given some medication to sedate me a bit and sat in the chair trying to fight it while talking to them. I don't really remember too much after that. I said my goodbyes and got on the trolley. Eventually, I was taken down to theatre at around 7:15 A.M. I vaguely remember the anaesthetist explaining what was happening, then it was lights out and I fell asleep.

I was in theatre for twelve hours in total. I understand the nurses called Tracey and Mum three times throughout the day with updates on my progress from the surgical team. They got the final call around 9:30 P.M. to say that I was out of surgery and now in ICU. The operation had gone well and they had removed the entire tumour. I'd also been given the heated chemotherapy (HIPEC) washout that kills all the microscopic cells. This treatment would continue for another four days after the operation. Due to the complexity of the operation, I was also given a temporary stoma that I'd need for approximately three months. This was to allow the bowel to rest and recover from the trauma of the operation.

My first memories after the operation are vague and very blurred. I remember the consultant telling me that I was out of theatre and the operation had gone well. He then went off to find my family and I soon fell asleep again.

I was sedated throughout the remainder of that night and was finally brought around the following morning. This time, both Tracey and Mum were there, but I was still intubated at this point so couldn't talk. I kept trying to tell them that I was cold. In the end, I was forced to write it down, and eventually after several attempts they understood and I was given an extra blanket.

The next time I woke, my breathing tube had been taken out and I was far more aware of my surroundings. I was still connected to various machines, including a nasogastric tube, a central line in my neck, an epidural, a PCA to administer morphine, two chest drains, six stomach drains and a catheter. I couldn't move without help from two nurses. I wasn't in too much pain but used my PCA to administer the morphine as and when I needed it. The epidural worked well, making me numb from the chest down. I was also given Ketamine, which had the effect of inducing hallucinations, which didn't start off too bad – just silly things such as mosquitoes flying around and the illusion of mice in the roof space – but some turned nasty.

I suffered auditory hallucinations to begin with and heard voices when no one was there. On the third night, I went through what seemed like a long and detailed hallucination, where I was dying. I saw vividly that I hadn't made it and I wasn't going to pull through. My family were brought in and I started saying my goodbyes and said I was sorry to be leaving them. It was all very real and I still struggle to think about it now. This really affected me in a bad way. The final two incidents were when I woke up and for a while didn't know who I was, or where or why I was there. Again it was all very strange, very disturbing.

A week passed and I was making good progress, when doctors started to talk about moving me out of ICU and into the High Dependency Ward. This really pleased me as I'd become tired of the ICU and knew the move was a step closer to getting home. Quite suddenly one evening, it was announced I was moving and staff arrived to carefully transport me to the specialist ward. I'd hoped for a single room again and was disappointed to find that I would be sharing the room with another patient. My first thought was that I hoped he didn't snore. It took me a while to settle; I was a little unnerved by the fact that I no longer received the one-to-one attention of a nurse around the clock. However, the environment was quieter and there was more space for my visitors.

I introduced myself to my room-mate. His name was Ron, a lovely old fellow well into his eighties. We started with all the usual questions about each other – where we lived, family, kids, all that kind of thing.

'What line of work did you do?' I enquired.

'You don't want to know that while you're in here, mate,' Ron replied.

'Yeah, sure I do,' I said.

'I was an undertaker,' he said, smiling.

I found this very funny and we both had a good laugh about it, instantly becoming best of friends. I spent just over a week sharing the room with Ron, never running out of things to chat about.

Outside, the weather was cold and snow showers blew through regularly. As each day passed, I gradually improved and grew stronger. I started walking further with the help of the physiotherapist. Soon I could walk on my own, once all the drips, drains and various tubes had been removed.

Living with the stoma wasn't an issue, contrary to what I had imagined. I'd become quite proficient at emptying, cleaning and changing the bag. This was my last hurdle to overcome, and the following day I was told I could go home. My clothes literally hung off me; I'd lost over two stone in the time I'd been in hospital.

The two-hour journey home was a long one and I was exhausted by the time we arrived. It was a tearful reunion but at least I was home; I'd actually made it. The following few weeks, I continued with daily walks and gradually grew stronger and stronger. Adapting to home life, living with a stoma and coming to terms with what I had been through was a struggle, but at least I was getting better.

Three months passed, and I went back to Basingstoke Hospital to have my stoma reversal operation. The operation was a walk in the park compared to the MOAS and all went well. Afterwards, I did have a rough time though and was quite ill for two or three days before my bowels started working properly again. I remember quite clearly sitting outside the hospital reception one evening, in my dressing gown, watching the sunset with my arm around Tracey. We took in the fresh air and for the first time I felt like a normal person again. I was truly starting to feel better.

I spent a few more weeks at home recovering and then finally returned to work. Initially, I started off working just half days then built up to full-time. It was great to get back into my busy life again and not have the worry of my operation and cancer hanging over my head.

While in Basingstoke for the stoma reversal, I'd decided I wanted to try to raise some money for the PMP ward. This would allow them to continue their research into this rare form of cancer. So I soon found myself planning a sponsored walk around the Snowdon Horseshoe. We would take in the ridges around each side of the mountain as well as the peak itself. I was joined by other friends and family, including a fellow PMP sufferer who had endured the MOAS operation at the Christie Hospital in Manchester and was raising money for them. It was great that both specialist centres in the UK would benefit from the one event. It was only six months since my MOAS and three months since my stoma reversal. We had a great day, completing the walk in around seven hours, and we raised thousands of pounds for both the hospitals.

A MOTHER'S PERSPECTIVE

MEMBERSHIP: # 18

Alessandro kept vomiting for nearly a week so I decided it was best to take him to the doctor. Their opinion was he simply had a stomach infection, but he didn't get any better. Therefore, a week later, I took him to the hospital and this time they thought he had hepatitis. However, when they did an ultrasound, they soon discovered he had a large tumour, which measured about 7 cm by 10 cm in size.

He was immediately hospitalized on the Saturday, and by Wednesday morning we had been rushed to England from Gibraltar, where we lived. I have two other children, both girls, aged one and ten years old. Alessandro is the oldest at eleven years old.

Alessandro had now become very weak and looked almost yellow; all he did was sleep. Initially, doctors thought the cancer was in his liver so we were transferred to a different hospital. Alessandro was actually put on a brand-new children's ward. As he was one of the first to be admitted to the new hospital, they gave him a commemorative certificate.

Surgeons were unable to operate because his tumour was so large it was pushing on his stomach, liver and heart. They felt such an operation would be way too risky and life-threatening. It was therefore decided his only chance was some very aggressive chemotherapy. I was told if this didn't work, there was very little else they could do to save him. I was obviously terrified at the thought of losing him.

He was to have chemotherapy every day for a whole week, and then once a week during the treatment he would go into theatre to also have it injected into his spine. When I arrived at the hospital one day, I remember seeing lots of other terribly sick children on the ward. One child had only just celebrated her first birthday; it was heart-wrenching and so sad. Alessandro thankfully slept most of the time during the first two months of his treatment. He had a very special teddy bear he took everywhere with him. He was so ill one night I thought he was going to die.

I spent the whole night with him, wondering whether I should keep the teddy as a reminder of Alessandro or bury it with him. My thinking was that at least he wouldn't be alone; he'd have his teddy he loved so much. As you can well imagine, this was an absolutely terrifying and worrying night.

One day, he shocked me by actually asking if he was going to die. He said he wondered because whatever computer game he'd asked for recently, I'd bought him. If truth be known, I really did think his time was limited so I didn't want him to go without anything, for what time he had left. I didn't normally spoil him but this was different. I obviously reassured him that he'd be fine and not die.

He made a lot of friends with other children on the ward and I formed some close friendships with their parents. It was just nice to talk and swap stories; this really helped us all a lot.

Alessandro was always the first in the classroom at the hospital, as thankfully he wanted to keep up with his schoolwork. One day, when he was too weak to go to school, the teachers gave him a musical keyboard, so he could keep himself occupied. Up until then, he'd never really listened to or shown any interest in music.

It was his sister who enjoyed music more. She was even having piano lessons. Alessandro had never been interested, but out of the blue one day he asked me what song I liked. The first thing that sprang to mind was the theme tune from *Titanic*; I didn't think any more of it. A few days later, he amazed me when he'd actually learnt how to play it on his keyboard. He played the whole tune to me really well, causing me to shed a few more tears, but this time they were tears of joy and happiness.

Thankfully, his chemotherapy went really well, and after seven months we were able to go back home to Gibraltar. I was so pleased as I was missing my daughters and had missed out on my youngest taking her first steps.

On the plane back, I explained to Alessandro that in Gibraltar it's quite unusual for children to have cancer and some kids might make fun of him due to him losing his hair. Thankfully, he said, 'It's their problem, not mine.'

He really made me feel so proud of the way he dealt with the whole situation at such a young age. As soon as we arrived back, instead of going home, he wanted to go straight to school; this was a first. He was so keen to see all his friends and teachers who'd supported us while we'd been away. Alessandro had spent his twelfth birthday in England and his school friends had made him a lovely birthday card. His attitude had always been strong and positive and, although he doesn't remember much about England, we made some very good friends while we were there.

As soon as I could, I arranged for him to have piano lessons as I wanted him to be able to read music properly, even though he was already playing songs using his PlayStation. Alessandro started his lessons just five years ago and has already completed stage six, which he passed with distinctions; there are only eight stages in total. He's entered local competitions and has always come away with a prize. Last year, he won the top award for the competition of 'Young Musician of the Year' sponsored by Albert Hammond, the famous songwriter. Alessandro actually composed the winning song himself. He has written a total of nine songs and has also played in various restaurants, hotels and pubs.

He is now seventeen and is a very noble and good kid, not your normal teenager. He even helps around the house and is an A student in school. Alessandro is currently studying music for his A-levels and wants to go to a music university in London to further his studies.

He never really likes to talk about his cancer or the treatment; he just says that it was his past and it's his future that he's concerned about. His view on life is to just get on with it and leave the past where it belongs. He now wakes up playing the piano and sleeps after playing the piano. Music is his whole life, and who knows, maybe if he hadn't got cancer, we would never have discovered his natural hidden talent.

Not long after this story was sent to me, 'Mrs Metcalfe' asked that I change both her and her son's name for privacy reasons; however, she was exceptionally happy for her story to be published in the hope it helps others.

HOW IT WAS

MEMBERSHIP: # 19

I was a young, fit fifty-one year old when I found a lump in my breast. I'd had lumps before, but, thankfully, after seeing a specialist and having mammograms, they always turned out to be cysts. This lump appeared during a very hectic time in my life. With help from other relatives, I was looking after my elderly parents, so this was a physically and emotionally busy time. Both my parents were very poorly. Sadly, in March, we regretfully decided they needed more professional and experienced residential care.

On the Friday, they were both admitted to a care home, and I thought, 'Right, on Monday, I'm going to see the doctor and get my lump checked out.' My doctor quickly referred me to the hospital and just two days later I went through a number of tests and examinations. I also had a mammogram, scan and a biopsy taken. I was still busy, just in a different way. Once all the tests were completed, the consultant called me back into his office and said those dreaded words: 'Yes, it is cancer.' He might as well have hit me with a sledgehammer; I was totally knocked over by the news.

'You knew, didn't you?' he asked.

I suppose deep down I did wonder, but chose to believe it wasn't anything more than another cyst. I'd had the lump for several months and knew I should have seen my doctor sooner. However, due to previous test results always coming back clear and my time being occupied looking after my parents, I'd chosen the easier option. I talked things through with the consultant, and another appointment was made for the following Tuesday.

This gave me time to digest the news and think about the options I'd been given, including having a mastectomy. I felt way too young and healthy to have my breast partially or even completely removed.

In the meantime, I carried on throwing myself into my work and dancing. I was a dance teacher for children and adults with learning difficulties and special needs. As well as this, I also ran a book-keeping business so always kept very busy.

3 April – It was my birthday but I obviously felt I didn't have too much to celebrate. I did have two lovely cats, though: Mitzi and Pixie.

Mitzi was pregnant and due to have kittens at any time, so I decided to visit the vet and find out if it was likely she would have them while I was in hospital. I was told the kittens could be here any day and it looked like there would be four of them. I explained I was going into hospital and was hoping they'd arrive once I got home. 'You'll be lucky,' the vet said.

Once home, I told Mitzi to hold on until I was discharged, but wasn't convinced she understood me. She seemed more interested in having a brush.

My next appointment was at the Breast Care Centre where I told the consultant that, after a lot of thinking and sleepless nights, I'd made the decision to go ahead with the mastectomy. He was delighted and thought it was the right decision for my long-term health. He explained my breast cancer was stage two: small and hormone related. He also said the operation would be done the following week. I was pleased with this – the sooner the better from my perspective. I just wanted to get it over with. I explained to the consultant that I didn't want the chemotherapy, radiotherapy or any reconstructive surgery.

His response was that I might still need to have it, despite having the breast removed. However, they wouldn't know for sure until after the operation.

I was booked to have my breast removed on 12 April. My stay in hospital would be for about five days and it would take another eight or so weeks at home to recover fully. I'd also not be able to drive for four weeks; this was going to be a big hindrance. In the big picture, I guess not driving was the least of my troubles. I remember the doctor started to explain what would happen after my stay in hospital, but I stopped him. 'Nope, just one step at a time please,' I said. I needed to deal with my cancer slowly, in my own way.

As soon as I got home I started making plans for my stay in hospital and continued telling Mitzi to hold off having her kittens until I was back. I told her every day. I still wasn't sure she was listening – like most cats she was more interested in her food.

12 April – A lady called Margaret whom I met while in hospital was going to be there at the same time as me. We first met while I was waiting to hear my test results. We soon got chatting and found we had so much in common.

My friend Teresa came with me to the hospital. When we arrived, I immediately noticed Margaret; she had some relatives keeping her company. We all sat together and Margaret and I were told by the nurses not to drink anything after 10:00 A.M. We were all joking about, pretending we were at an airport lounge waiting to be transported to some exotic destination. This helped pass the time and made us both feel a little more relaxed. At 10:15 A.M., we were called in, first Margaret and then me.

We laughed with the receptionist about being in an airport lounge and she joined in the fun; either that or she thought we were absolutely mad. We completed the necessary paperwork and were given instructions on how to find the ward. 'You can wait there for your flight,' the nurse joked.

As we entered the ward, we continued doing our best to keep our spirits up; again, we tried to forget how nervous we were now feeling. We told the staff how we were imagining we were going on a sun-drenched holiday. The nurse showed us to the 'airport lounge' and told us the stewardess would be with us shortly.

Soon, I was lying on a hospital bed being whisked off to theatre with the porter, nurse and Teresa pushing. The joking had stopped now and I was starting to feel very anxious indeed. We arrived at the theatre, where I was moved onto another bed, then Teresa and I said our goodbyes before she went home. When the various consultants, anaesthetists and other doctors greeted me and asked how I was, I replied, 'Suddenly nervous.' They all did their best to reassure me everything would be OK.

The next thing I knew, it was midnight, my breast had been removed and I just remember my throat feeling really dry.

13 April (Good Friday) – I was given a cup of tea and a bed pan. When a nurse came around to change my dressing, I asked if I could see my scar. The nurse said, 'Really, are you ready?' I nodded; the sooner the better, I thought. The nurse slowly uncovered the site and let me take a quick peek at where my right breast had been. Once I'd seen the scar, my fears instantly dispersed; I was so pleased I'd asked.

If I'd hung on and waited a few more days, the dread would have built up inside me.

My friend Margaret was in the next bed to me, which was nice as we were able to chat and look after each other.

Later that day, I managed to walk to the toilet with the help of the staff and even managed to wash myself. The staff kept a close eye on me as I got back into bed, just in case I fell. I was told I'd be able to get dressed the following day. I also had a number of visitors, which was really nice.

14 April – I got myself washed and dressed without the nurse's help, which I was so pleased about. I put my big comfy jumper on and managed to stuff the various tubes and bag under it. I kept telling other patients I was six months pregnant and it wouldn't be long before my baby arrived. If nothing else, I'd convinced them I was mad! It's always good to keep a sense of humour in these situations, even if it was only me laughing.

15 April (Easter Sunday) – I had lots of visitors, which really helped the time pass. I even managed to walk down

to the café for a drink. I was so looking forward to getting home now and seeing my cats. I kept my fingers crossed Mitzi hadn't had her kittens yet.

16 April (Easter Monday) – I had a steady flow of visitors again and the tube in my hand and the drain in my chest were removed. The painkillers were too strong for me now, so I decided just to have some paracetamol.

17 April – I asked the consultant if I could go home and explained about Mitzi being pregnant.

He agreed, and after arranging the paperwork I finally got home.

18 April – At 3:00 A.M., Teresa and I watched Mitzi deliver her kittens. She really had been listening to me. She had five kittens in total: two black and white, which looked a little like her; two grey and white; and one pure grey. This was a big boost to my recovery and perfect timing, too.

19 April – I had to go back to the hospital to see what they had found during my operation. I was told the cancer had spread to my lymph glands and they had therefore removed them. Because of this, it was decided I would need some chemotherapy and radiotherapy. I felt very numb at the news and started doing things in a complete daze, knowing I'd need more treatment. I guess I'd hoped by having the mastectomy all the cancerous cells would have been removed. My dear Mitzi and her kittens were so lovely and really helped to take my mind off the situation but I knew I still had some big decisions to make.

1 May – My appointment with Oncology arrived, confirming I'd need both chemotherapy and radiotherapy. I continued to recover from my operation, while disbelieving I'd need

further treatment. This was another nightmare I didn't want either. My niece visited me and brought some books about breast cancer, as well as information on the 'Bristol Approach' published by the Penny Brohn Cancer Centre. This centre was started by Penny Brohn, along with Pat Pilkington, who wanted to develop a holistic programme for people with cancer. As I started to read it, the more I wanted to find out.

14 May – At my appointment with the oncologist, I gave her a list of my allergies and told her what reactions I have to certain things. She told me that the chemotherapy would be more life-threatening than the actual cancer because of all my allergies. She explained that she wanted me to have radiotherapy because it would give me a seventy percent chance of the breast cancer not returning; obviously, I agreed. I explained I was taking Arimidex and some strong painkillers, but was having a lot of side effects. She advised I stop taking the Arimidex for a while.

When I saw my doctor a few days later, he also suggested I stop taking painkillers. This meant I could only take paracetamol. As I'd stopped the painkillers, I decided it was time to try a little meditation and some relaxation exercises. I'd been doing exercises since the operation to help with my arm and shoulder, and was almost able to straighten it above my head.

18 May – I was now able to drive again; only a short distance, but I really felt like I was making progress. When the post arrived that morning, I opened an envelope to see a list of dates for my radiotherapy sessions, which was really scary. Feeling concerned, I phoned the helpline and they talked me through what was involved. They even suggested I visit them before I start my treatment, to see the machines. When I put

the phone down, I cried bucketloads; it felt as though all the emotion and shock of having breast cancer had suddenly found its way out. I was on my own and knew I didn't want the radiotherapy but realized I had to have it; I felt trapped. I also had to have an MRI scan at the end of the month; this terrified me, too. I used to have a real problem in confined spaces and this fear was returning. I had coped well with the surgery and my stay in hospital, but the radiotherapy really worried me. I no longer felt the brave person I'd been up to now. At 7:00 P.M., I spoke with the radiotherapy helpline again. The nurse was lovely and we chatted for well over half an hour. She explained how important the radiotherapy was for me, which helped calm my nerves.

19 May – Saturday again; the weeks were flying past, even though I wasn't working. The kittens were already trying to get out of their box; eventually, it was the smallest one that managed it first. By the end of the day, they were all running about on the floor. They were such a tonic and really helped to cheer me up.

21 May – My niece took me to the Oncology Department and help centre to talk about my forthcoming radiotherapy. The lady I met was very helpful and showed me photos of the machines to alleviate my fears.

29 May – I sat in the waiting room looking at the other people, wondering if they were waiting to see the consultant to find out if they had breast cancer. I wanted to say, 'It's OK, everything will be all right; it's not as bad as you think.' When I was talking to the nurse, she asked if she could give out my telephone number to a few people who had just been diagnosed, who were waiting for their operation. I immediately

said, 'Yes.' If I could help anyone, I was more than pleased to do so. That evening, my niece drove me to the relaxation centre, where I did some meditation and healing, which I found really helped me.

30 May – I visited the Oncology Department to have my MRI scan, which I'd not been looking forward to one bit. Thankfully, Teresa came with me for support, which helped. I took one of my favourite music CDs to try to help relax me.

When I was called, I explained I was claustrophobic and extremely nervous. The staff were all lovely and so understanding; they made me feel more relaxed and comfortable. I climbed onto the bed with the machine above my body. They measured me, drew lines over my right breast area where I'd had the operation and demonstrated how the machine would come down close to my body. They explained that the machine would make a noise for several minutes and then it would stop and then start again; this would happen three times. They said I could ask them to stop at any time, but it would obviously take longer as they'd have to start from the beginning. They played my music and talked to me all the time through headphones while I was being scanned. In my mind, I managed to turn the noise the machine made into the sea, waves crashing against the sea walls. On the final section, I was actually visualizing standing on a beach with my friends in a circle around me. We were all drumming and I was dancing. I found this helped me to get through it, by visualizing something much nicer. Once the MRI had finished, the noise stopped and the machine was lifted up away from me. I needed to stay there a little longer while they took photos of the pen marks on me. They couldn't use the normal type of pens they used on other people because of my allergies. This meant the marks might get washed off in the shower. The pen marks would show them the exact place to give me the radiotherapy each time. They gave me a marker pen and asked me to renew the lines each time I showered until the radiotherapy was complete, or until the tattoo marks could be made.

I got myself dressed, and before I left a radiographer took Teresa and me along to the simulator room to show me where I'd go the following week for my radiotherapy.

When we got outside, the relief was so massive I burst out crying. Teresa gave me a reassuring hug and we headed off to find somewhere nice outside in the sun for lunch. Afterwards, I felt much better and was pleased how well I'd coped. If you're reading this and you suffer from claustrophobia, I can assure you it's not that bad – if I can do it, so can you.

9 June – I had a lovely relaxing weekend in Minehead, enjoying the company of friends and beautiful sea views and walks. It was just what I needed before I began my radiotherapy treatment.

18 June – The day had come to start my radiotherapy. I was to receive four minutes per day, five days a week. I was due to have four weeks like this and on the fifth and final week finish with a double dose. After the tenth day, I was feeling really ill with my allergies, so arranged to see a doctor. I told her I wasn't sure I could go through with any more radiotherapy treatment. She told me that, while she understood it was hard for me, I must continue. I came away feeling even more upset than when I arrived.

Over the weekend, I decided I needed to take a break from the treatment and phoned Oncology on the Monday. They told me the machines were broken, but would be fixed by Tuesday, when I must come in.

On Tuesday morning, I phoned the Radiotherapy Department again and said I couldn't make it. They told me that this was the last day I could have off without it affecting my treatment. I was told if I cancelled any more appointments I would have to start the course again. They reminded me that, if I continued with the treatment, I would have a seventy percent chance of not getting breast cancer again. However, if I missed any more sessions, the treatments I'd had already wouldn't be effective and it would have been a waste of time.

This was the hardest decision I've ever had to make in my whole life. I needed to make sure I was doing the right thing. I phoned the Penny Brohn Cancer Centre. They obviously could not advise me but suggested I read a book called *Your Life in Your Hands*. I had already tried to find information about stopping the radiotherapy halfway through, without any success. Coincidentally, I already owned the book, so sat down and read it the whole way through. I then did some meditation for a while and came to the decision that I was going to stop having radiotherapy. I kept asking myself what if I was wrong. I sat down in the kitchen and wrote a list of reasons for stopping and soon became convinced my decision to stop was the right one.

During the next few days, I decided I would attend some of the Penny Brohn Cancer Centre courses. I saw my doctor as I knew I'd need his approval and some forms signing. I explained about stopping the radiotherapy and he said I was one patient who knew my body better than anyone. He felt sure I'd done the right thing for me. In fact, he suggested that I contact the Penny Brohn Cancer Centre, and I said, 'Well, you won't mind signing these then,' and presented him with their forms.

18 July – I got myself measured up for my prosthesis. When I saw what they looked like, I was so relieved and pleased that it was small, soft and light. I had expected it to be heavy as they used to be years ago. I then went shopping for some new bras with a pocket for my prosthesis and got home feeling invigorated and like a new person. I was now on my way to feeling more confident and looking forward to the future.

It took me two years before I could go back to work, which was mainly due to the difficulties I'd had with the radiotherapy treatments and my allergies. During the two years I was at home, I carried on working on my self-development, which was proving very worthwhile. I read loads of self-help books, received art therapy, healing, reflexology and other alternative therapies from the guys at the Penny Brohn Cancer Centre. I'd always been interested in alternative medicine, and the cancer centre courses and healing really aided my recovery.

Six years after my operation, I'm pleased to say my consultant shook my hand recently and said, 'You did know your body and knew what was right for you – congratulations.'

I am still working full-time as an accounts manager, colour counsellor, healer, teacher and colour life coach; I love keeping busy. I also like supporting people with breast cancer on the www.CancerInCommon.com online forum.

Finally, I have now been completely discharged from the breast care centre after my mammogram in April.

I want to thank everyone who has helped me, especially my family, Margaret and Teresa, Mitzi and Pixie, my doctor and consultant, and all the staff at the Penny Brohn Cancer Centre.

SALIVA, CHOPPED PORK AND DIVORCE

MEMBERSHIP: # 1

I was encouraged but not surprised to read that scientists have developed a breath test, which detects cancer before patients suffer any symptoms. I say I'm not surprised because for years the police have been able to detect the vintage of the wine I've been drinking, by my simply blowing into a bag. In fact, by looking at a swab of my saliva, doctors can obtain my DNA and work out who my ancestors were. Not wanting to show off, but just one whiff of my wife's breath in the morning and I can detect what she had for dinner the previous night. Actually, best I change the subject – divorce comes to mind.

I had one reader email me, asking if I'd explain in detail the medical terminology I use. So, for her benefit and wanting to prove I listen to my readers – a little like David Cameron listening to his electorate – here goes. Saliva is a clear liquid secreted into the mouth by salivary glands and mucous glands; it moistens the mouth and starts the digestion of starches. Divorce is the legal dissolution of a marriage. Hope that makes sense, Mrs Copper?

With the ability to identify and learn so much about us just by poking around in our mouths, I'm surprised credit card companies haven't got us licking a machine when shopping. Forget 'Chip and Pin', how about 'Lick and Pay'? I might write to Barclaycard with my suggestion. Since DNA is unique, credit card companies could soon identify us and save the consumer from remembering yet another pin number or password.

Again for the benefit of Mrs Copper – DNA is a nucleic acid that contains genetic instructions used in the development and functioning of all known living organisms and viruses. Please, Mrs Copper – don't confuse this with a computer virus, like you confused junk email (Spam) with chopped pork and luncheon meat.

These scientists have developed sensors that can spot chemical signs of lung, breast, bowel and prostate cancer in a person's breath. They believe further work could lead to a cheap, portable 'electronic nose' capable of diagnosing cancer at an early stage. Now I'm not sure I'd be capable of that. My wife's previously eaten tofu is about my limit.

A team of scientists carried out tests on 177 volunteers, some healthy and others with different types of cancer. This study showed that an 'electronic nose' can distinguish between healthy and malignant breath. It can also differentiate between the breath of patients with different cancer types. If this is true, it could save millions of lives.

So, if your nasal senses aren't as efficient as mine, or until this 'electronic nose' is launched, do me a favour please – go and see your doctor if you feel unwell or notice any unusual lumps or bumps; feel free to blame me.

KEEP SMILING

MEMBERSHIP: # 20

At the age of fifteen, I'd been diagnosed with diabetes, the sort that needed daily injections. I also needed a carefully controlled diet. Not ideal when I was experiencing the usual teenage problems; I'd just discovered girls. Despite the setback, I got on with living my life. I left school, got a job, then another, and eventually managed to keep a girlfriend for longer than five minutes.

To move the story forward, things appeared to be going well. Now in my late twenties, I'd got engaged to Sharon and eventually got a job that I enjoyed. I was still also managing to keep my diabetes under control.

Unfortunately, out of the blue one day, I fainted. I then continued to have fainting spells regularly and felt quite unwell. After several fainting episodes, Sharon convinced me to see my doctor. After explaining my symptoms, it was naturally thought diabetes was the cause of my problems. He decided to refer me to one of the diabetes specialists for further tests.

Two weeks passed and, despite looking after myself a little better as the specialists had suggested, I started to feel even worse. I had also now developed a rash so went back to see my doctor again. I saw a different doctor this time, as my usual doctor was away. He examined me, checked my eyes and looked at the rash. His thoughts were that it might not actually be the diabetes causing the problems, and he made an appointment for me to visit the Haematology Unit the following day. I remember the appointment quite vividly.

After the tests and a very painful procedure with a large needle, I was told I'd need to stay overnight at the hospital. They neglected to mention that I had Acute Myeloid Leukaemia, which I didn't find out until I was ushered into an isolation room; oh, and asked to sign some consent forms.

How to explain the story now is difficult, as the chances are most people reading this will be familiar with the usual side effects some cancer treatments can cause.

These included hair loss, which for me was a struggle as I loved my long hair. I had big hair, think Duran Duran style, sad but true! Other problems included trouble sleeping, poor concentration levels and having a Hickman line fitted.

I was also worried about the stress and upset I was causing my family and friends. I was very concerned by the awful news that the treatment would make it unlikely that Sharon and I would be able to have a family. Within just two hours of receiving this devastating news, I was asked to produce a sperm sample for storage. Having to retreat to the hospital en suite shower room to fill a plastic pot was far from appealing. I wish I could say I was successful and filled it to the top; however, with all the will in the world, the romance was missing – nothing happened.

Anyway, for six weeks, I lay in bed having treatment. My hair started to fall out, which was making me resemble Buster from Bad Manners. I had drips bleeping away and my wee being measured out in cardboard cups. Sharon sat with me every day and did her best to keep me going. We had some very funny moments together, which really helped me get through my treatment.

Once, the television in the corner of my hospital room was so loud it made it difficult for us both to actually hear each other. The theme tune from *Top Gear* was blasting out. Spontaneously, both Sharon and I started playing our air guitars and hummed for all we were worth, only stopping when the laughing got so loud. The nursing staff came rushing in thinking I was crying with pain; they didn't believe me when I said they were tears of laughter.

Eventually, my treatment was reduced and I was allowed home. I still had to come into hospital daily; unfortunately, at that time, our car was proving very unreliable and it finally broke down on the way in one morning. A breakdown driver soon arrived in the dirtiest truck imaginable and said he'd have to take our car to a garage; all I was concerned about was all the germs. I still had to be careful as my immune system was low after all my treatment, making me very prone to infection. Anyway, I had no choice so asked if he could drop me off at the hospital. On the way, we started talking about my cancer and the various treatments. As we pulled up to the hospital, he said a friend of his brother had the same but had died, 'which was sad because he was a good customer'. Not really a story I wanted to hear at that point.

There is humour to be found in most situations and I always felt it was important to allow myself to laugh. Sometimes it helped me to cry and scream; in fact, being selfish at times helped me, too. I hoped everyone understood it wasn't personal.

To bring my story to an end, I am now happily married to the lovely Sharon and we have a son and daughter conceived naturally with no need for test tubes or plastic pots. I also now work full-time at a college.

There are still times when I worry or get depressed, but I only have to think back and realize the worst is behind me. So, if you're reading this going through treatment or getting over cancer, stay positive and live your life to the full. It can and will get better, and remember you are not alone, people like me are thinking of you.

TOO FRIGHTENED TO ASK

MEMBERSHIP: # 21

I was born in 1958 and raised in a town called Prudhoe in Northumberland. I have two brothers and a sister. My dad is still alive but unfortunately my mum died nine years ago from lung cancer.

My illness originally came to light in 1981 with the appearance of a lump on the right side of my neck. It was the size of an egg and I was able to move it about as it didn't hurt. It caused absolutely no pain or discomfort until one morning in August. I got up and told Mum it had started to feel very painful. She instantly sent me off to see the doctor. It was suggested I visit my dentist, who initially thought it was one of my wisdom teeth coming through. After an x-ray, the dentist sent me to a dental hospital; again, nothing could be found.

My doctor, after re-examining me, couldn't find anything either so suggested I have yet more x-rays. However, this time, they were going to inject a liquid into the lump, which would improve the image on the x-ray. Hopefully, this would allow them to see more. They put a needle attached to a tube into the saliva duct in my cheek. Doctors then pumped iodine into my neck and took images of my neck, throat and nose. This whole procedure took around an hour but felt much longer.

In October, I went to see a consultant with my mum. I was told they still didn't know what the lump was or what was causing it. We were asked to go along to Newcastle General Hospital for a biopsy to be taken. My appointment was in January of the following year. At the time, I was working as a domestic assistant at a hospital for the mentally handicapped.

I told my boss I was being admitted to hospital on Tuesday for a biopsy. I explained that I would have my operation Wednesday, recover Thursday and be home Friday. This would mean I'd be back at work the following Monday.

Anyway, I ended up staying in hospital for two weeks. They removed the lump and found one of my lymph glands was blocked. After a few days, they did a biopsy on my ears. The second week, they did another biopsy but this time taken from my nose.

I was never told the outcome of any of the biopsy results and I never thought to ask; but I was still very young at the time and left this to my mum.

On leaving the hospital, I was given an appointment to meet with the consultant a few weeks later, and both Mum and Dad came with me this time. The consultant explained I needed some radiotherapy but, before they could do this, all my teeth would need to be removed. It was explained that the radiotherapy would rot my teeth and they would eventually fall out anyway.

At this stage, I still didn't have any idea what was wrong with me. The shock of being in hospital and the news about the radiotherapy had caused my mind to go completely blank. I'd forgotten to ask – I know this sounds crazy. I just went along with everything I was told, as I trusted Mum and Dad and they appeared to understand the situation. I went back into hospital in February and on the Monday morning I was taken to theatre where all my teeth were removed, including my wisdom teeth.

At visiting time on Monday evening, my parents and a couple of their friends visited me. I was still feeling pretty groggy and my gums were bleeding. Dad gave me a package with 'Get Well' written on it. On opening it, I was gob-smacked – excuse the pun – to see it contained a family-size bag of salted peanuts. He looked at me and said, 'Something to enjoy when you get your new teeth.'

The ward sister thought it was a bit cruel to start with, but eventually saw it was a joke, done simply to try to cheer me up, and it worked.

The next day, I was measured up for a mask. It was made in two halves; the back was made first then the front. This was to protect my nose and other parts of my face from the radiotherapy. The day after the mask was measured, I was allowed home. We had an Alsatian dog called Major and when I got home he followed me everywhere. If I got up to make a cup of tea, he would be right beside me. If I went to the toilet he'd sit outside, and if I had a bath he would cry and scratch at the door until I let him in. When I mentioned to Mum I couldn't move without him being there, she said he obviously sensed I wasn't well and was trying to protect me. It's amazing what animals can pick up on.

A few weeks later, my radiotherapy started. I had to have it five days a week for four weeks. I felt a bit like a monster wearing my mask. The back half was screwed to the table and the front half was then put over my face and fitted to the back half with screws, preventing me from moving my head. A syringe was then put through a space round my mouth for me to breathe through. It was awful, and I felt very claustrophobic. On top of the mask, lead blocks were placed from my chin down so my throat wasn't affected by the radiotherapy. Stupidly, I still had no idea what was wrong with me. I must have been in denial or just a very ignorant young girl.

I wasn't allowed to wash my face or neck while having the radiotherapy for a further four weeks afterwards. I was only allowed to use talcum powder. Mum used to wash my hair over the bathroom sink. After each session, I would go home and have a sleep, then I'd get ready to go out for a few drinks and a game of bingo.

I wasn't a pretty sight travelling on the bus five nights a week to have an evening out with my friends; but I didn't care. If people didn't like seeing someone with no teeth, scabs and a spotty face, they could always look the other way, I thought. I knew whatever was wrong with me wouldn't last forever. Eventually, my treatment came to an end. I was worn out but it didn't stop me going out and trying to enjoy myself. Major still continued to follow me around the house like my shadow, bless him.

I got my new teeth fitted in August; they felt very strange at first and I really struggled to get used to them. They kept falling out whenever I ate; I also felt as if everyone was looking at me all the time. I was more self-conscious about my new teeth than I was about my spots and scabs. I had to get used to them quickly, though, as I was due to go on holiday to Benidorm in September with some friends from work; a holiday that I was really in need of by now.

On returning from holiday, I went back to work. At last, everything in my life was starting to get back to normal. I got back into my routine of being a domestic assistant, a job I really loved.

The last couple of months of the year went by with no problems. I was visiting the hospital regularly for check-ups and everything was going fine.

My sister Carol had moved to Bristol with a friend of ours called Jane. Carol had split up with her boyfriend and needed help to run the flat, so asked if I would like to move in with her. I said yes instantly. A new start and a new life was just what I needed.

In the April, I moved in with them. I still didn't know exactly what my illness had been at this time.

Unknown to me, Mum had spoken with Carol on the phone and asked her if she could tell me what had been wrong with me. It transpires I'd had a form of cancer called Anaplastic Carcinoma, which was located in the back of my nose and throat. The news still didn't really sink in. Looking back, I must have been in denial or just plain stupid for not asking. Don't answer that!

I kept plodding on with my life as though nothing was

wrong with me, even though I was still having check-ups at the hospital every three months. These check-ups went to every six months and then eventually annually. Finally, they stopped totally and I was discharged.

Not long afterwards, I met a nice guy called Jerry. He was helping with a disco at a friend's twenty-first birthday party. We started seeing each other and after three weeks he moved in with me. In the February we got engaged and in May we got married. I remember after the wedding service and reception Mum whispered to me, 'Well, honey, you got your fairytale wedding.' It was a great day and the proudest and happiest day of my life – until December a couple of years later. This is when I gave birth to our son, Christopher, and suddenly my life was complete, or so I thought.

Jerry and I became grandparents to Liam. We also celebrated our silver wedding anniversary two years ago, which for us was more of an achievement than most!

GETTING THE GIST

MEMBERSHIP: # 22

My story actually starts around forty years ago. I began to experience problems with blood seeping into my bowel, resulting in black-coloured motions. I'm trying to be as polite as I can! Various tests were performed to try to identify the cause. These included an endoscopy, barium meals and a scan. However, no conclusive reason could be identified. This became a routine that repeated itself over the years. My problems appeared to possibly be associated with the consumption of spicy Oriental or Asian foods and drinking lager. It was recommended I limit my intake of alcohol and contact a specialist consultant if the symptoms reappeared.

As I was born in Scotland, where it is well known that the dietary culture leaves much to be desired, it occurred to a few doctors that there could well have been incidences of ulceration of my oesophagus or even my stomach tract while growing up.

There were repeat episodes over the following twenty-four years with further internal examinations, but still no cause could be found. But on almost all occasions, by the time I was examined, the bleeding had stopped. Each episode resulted in a fairly substantial loss of blood, causing considerable weakness and a lengthy recovery, even with medication. As a side issue, my doctor noticed my complaint regarding excessive acid reflux since I was a youngster. He thought I probably had lactose intolerance. He suggested at the time I should try changing to soya milk, which I did.

Amazingly, over two or three weeks, there was a marked reduction in the amount of times I suffered from excessive acid, which I was naturally pleased about. However, it didn't completely eradicate the bleeding into the bowel.

After a family get-together at Christmas, which included overeating and indulging in alcohol, albeit with lemonade mixed in it, I noticed that I had lost blood again. Within two hours of contacting my doctors, I found myself in hospital. However, I was only put into a ward for observation. By the time I was seen by a doctor, the bleeding had stopped completely.

The following day, I was seen by a consultant on his rounds with his junior doctors. They had a quick look at me and gave me a prod and poke, initially by the consultant who couldn't detect any abnormality in the stomach region and then by the juniors. They all came up with the same result, except one. A young African doctor indicated that he thought he could detect a mass and, after a short discussion with the consultant, who didn't agree, sent me off for an ultrasound scan. There it was: a large mass between the abdominal wall and my main organs.

I was informed after the scan that I was going to be moved to another hospital for further checks. Here it was confirmed that I had what was called Gastrointestinal Stromal Tumour (GIST); in other words, I had cancer. The news was a massive shock to both me and my family.

It transpired that the GIST tumour was quite rare. As it has several genetic variations, a biopsy was needed. This was done under a local anaesthetic on the hospital ward.

I was actually shown a colour image of the tumour on a screen by the doctor and remember thinking how fantastic technology is to see this. Being able to look at the growth pulsing inside me was almost like watching an alien species in a *Doctor Who* episode, but obviously much more worrying – unless you're a ten year old!

Some time elapsed before I could see the consultant who specialized in this particular condition. When I did, I was told that the tumour was an aggressive type and it measured about 12 cm by 5 cm. I was going to be given a course of Glivec chemotherapy tablets. It was hoped these would shrink the tumour over the next six to eight months.

I asked about the biopsy I'd had in February, but they still hadn't got any results back from the labs. They said they'd let me know as soon as they heard anything. It was during a later discussion regarding my progress in April that I was told they still didn't have the results back. On checking with the laboratory, it was discovered that they hadn't actually been sent away. I was so cross. We finally got the results in June and I did – as they originally thought – have GIST. I had the 'C Kit 9' gene, which worryingly wasn't responsive to the Glivec treatment. So I was now going to be given a treatment of Sunitinib. The bad news was this wasn't supported by the local NHS partnership as a first line of treatment.

I'd begun to take a herbal treatment recommended by a qualified herbalist who worked with both the university and several physicians.

She'd found the treatment to be very effective against many forms of cancer, and felt it would help improve my immune system in preparation for an operation in November to remove the tumour.

I discussed the operation with the surgeon during his clinic and he advised me that he was unable to confirm whether or not he would be able to perform micro-surgery, or full open surgery. He needed more time to examine the condition of the tumour, its size and position, and any potential obstacles around the area first.

Eventually, on 10 November, I had my operation. Afterwards, the surgeon informed me the tumour had been successfully removed, plus results from his tests proved that there was no trace of any other cancerous tissue around the area. Two days after the operation, I was seen by a physio-therapist who was surprised at my ability to walk a longer distance than she suggested. I was able to walk up and down two flights of stairs after just four days. She thought I'd be able to go home in just two more days. I put my fast recov-ery down to topping up my immune system with the herbal treatment. I was so grateful for the care shown to me by the ward staff, surgeon and his clinical nursing team.

On Sunday, I was back home being treated with loads of love and care from my family, particularly my eldest daughter Lisa, who also has a very strong belief in the benefit of herbal treatments. By the Tuesday of the following week, I was out walking fairly long distances. Sometimes I was a grumpy old 'wotsit' admittedly and found getting dressed and going to bed a little uncomfortable.

Today it is almost three years since I left hospital. I'm now enjoying life and think myself extremely fortunate that a young doctor whom I never saw again had the belief that he could sense that mass. Wherever he is, I give thanks to him almost every day.

A WEIGHTY PROBLEM

MEMBERSHIP: # 1

I have discovered that a newspaper columnist should avoid certain subjects. Mention religion, politics or people with ginger hair and my mailbox fills faster than a ferry to the UK when volcanic ash is in the air. So I know I'm on safe ground to highlight areas where the NHS could save some money.

Overweight people visit their doctor twelve percent more and spend nineteen percent more time in hospital. The average visit to a hospital costs you – the taxpayer – between £410 and £1,027, depending on whose report you believe.

So, with 463 patients being seen a minute, and with forty-three percent of men and thirty-three percent of women being overweight, I have found a great and obvious method of cutting our national debt – start charging the fat bastards. Before you start yelling, yes, I am qualified to make such a statement. I've lost six stone over four years, so genuinely appreciate how much willpower is required.

With this in mind, I fail to understand why our Chancellor of the Exchequer, George Osborne MP, or his assistant, the ginger-haired Chief Secretary Danny Alexander, doesn't create a 'Fat Tax'.

Why stop there? It costs you – the taxpayer – over £374 million a year in treating cirrhosis of the liver. So let's start charging some of the 15,200,000 people who attend Accident & Emergency each year, who have self-inflicted problems – such as alcohol poisoning or drug abuse. It's estimated the NHS spends £3 billion a year on alcohol abuse alone.

At this rate, I'm either going to be asked to be Mayor of Somerset or assassinated.

There are over 43,000 admissions to our hospitals attributed to thugs brawling. Let's charge them; if they can afford alcohol, they can afford a fine. The government doesn't hesitate to fine me just for doing 5 mph over the speed limit and I'm not costing anyone money. In fact, I'm using more petrol so providing additional revenue to the public purse in tax.

While I'm at it, let's charge for the anti-obesity treatments, such as drugs or gastric bands. The Department of Health says obesity will cost the NHS in England £6.3 billion a year by 2015. Forget Mayor – at this rate, I'll be the next Prime Minister.

Another reason my mates George and Dan should listen is because being overweight is linked to cancers like breast, prostate and ovarian. Cancer treatment is very expensive. Hazel Blears said, 'There are clear links between obesity and our biggest killers – heart disease and cancer.'

It seems ironic that the overweight, drug-taking alcoholics are given no-expense-spared help and assistance. Yet the old, ill and genuinely frail are not wanted clogging up our hospital beds. Should you be a cancer sufferer wanting unusual or expensive chemotherapy, you either have to pay for it yourself or create so much media attention your local authority backs down.

I'm so pleased I've managed to avoid any contentious subjects this week!

CANCER IS A WORD, NOT A SENTENCE

MEMBERSHIP: # 23

Just a couple of days before my daughter's third birthday in May, I was diagnosed with cancer: Non-Hodgkin Lymphoma (NHL). My son was then only months old. I was thirty-three and had no symptoms. In fact, I had never felt better in my life. My husband, like all good amorous men, went in for the 'cop a feel' one morning and felt a lump in my breast. I had no idea it was there. I thought nothing more of it, it was no big deal.

A couple of weeks passed and I had a general check-up. The doctor asked if I had any questions. I mentioned the lump and was sent for an ultrasound to rule anything out. Within thirty minutes of my seeing the sonographer, a second doctor was asked to take a look at my lump. The doctor ordered a fine-needle biopsy and found the lump very hard to penetrate. The first thing I thought of was breast cancer and I had no idea what was to follow. The next day, I was referred to an oncologist who bluntly told me it was serious and it needed to be dealt with and quickly. My NHL had presented itself outside the lymph system and the test results therefore showed it was a high-grade cancer. I immediately had surgery to remove the lump and started a six-month course of chemotherapy.

I was sent to the main hospital, which was an hour away from my family, as there was no available treatment for my type of cancer nearer to home. My blood was tested before the chemotherapy began. If all my blood counts were good, the chemotherapy could start. I was then moved to the Oncology Ward. I lovingly named it the 'Penthouse Suite' because it was situated on the top floor of the hospital. I was the youngest in the Penthouse Suite, which made me feel uncomfortable. I felt so isolated and out of place.

I would start the weekly routine with cancer-fighting drugs. The first week was the hardest. My husband and children were an hour away and I couldn't stop thinking I should be with them and not stuck in hospital. I felt so alone and afraid, and being miles from home didn't help. I was frightened of the unknown more than anything, my mind playing tricks with me. I knew people could die from cancer; I'd sadly met a few. I kept asking myself if I too was going to die from cancer; would this be my fate?

The nurses would enter my room, all gowned up, gloves on and looking as if they were entering a hazardous infected zone. I guess they were but it felt so hostile. I continued lying there in my nightie, wondering if I should also be wearing protective gear.

My husband brought the children to visit me a couple of times a week. It was so good to see them – oh, how I missed my babies. My daughter would look closely at the central line and watch the fluid being pumped into me. She asked so many questions; she wanted to know everything. She would hold my hand and look into my eyes. I could feel the love she had for me, and I struggled not to cry. Just the sight of her sadness was enough to make me determined to fight this terrible disease. When it was time for them to leave, I always felt so empty and alone and silently cried. Thoughts, crazy thoughts, would rush around my mind. In hindsight, my mind was playing tricks and I became my own worst enemy at times.

I never once thought anyone else could be going through what I was experiencing. It felt like I was the only one in the world with cancer.

I worried about not being with my children and missing their various milestones; this made me so angry. I was very upset and kept asking myself: 'Why me?' There was no history of cancer in our family. I was healthy and fit. I was a good person. I didn't deserve any of this; it just didn't feel fair. What had I ever done to deserve this? I thought about every little thing I could have done for hours. I yelled at my poor dad once when I was eight. I fought with my sisters while growing up. I may have even told the odd white lie. Was this my punishment, getting cancer?

There was nothing else to do in hospital but think, which certainly caused my mind to spin way too fast. The nurses were great and helped entertain me – and annoyed me at times, too. They would wake me throughout the night to give me chemotherapy, saline or just to take my blood pressure and temperature. I'd also be woken at four o'clock each morning and asked to stand on the scales. Why on earth did they want to weigh me at 4:00 A.M.? I became obsessed and recorded my weight, too. Some days I lost four pounds and other days I put weight on. I wanted to stay the same but it was impossible as I had no appetite.

Food made me feel ill and the smell was terrible. I couldn't eat much and yet I still managed to put weight on. The nurses could see I wasn't eating and mixed up a hospital protein drink, full of vitamins and minerals. Umm, delicious, not...

The drug treatment I was receiving was tough; it took a lot out of me. It was given in small doses but more frequently to minimize the side effects.

Unfortunately, it didn't minimize my hair loss. I'd always had long hair growing halfway down my back, which I loved. I was in the hospital bathroom when I noticed my hair falling out, not just a little, but lots, from everywhere. Michael, my husband, finally cut it short with some scissors. Then, a few days later, he went over it again with clippers as more clumps finally fell out. I remember standing next to my father with our matching *GI Jane* haircuts; it was actually very funny looking back. Within a day or two, I was totally bald – I'd lost all my hair. Eyelashes, brows and below, clean as a whistle, as some would say.

It took months to get used to not having hair, but at least it was painless. I felt as if everyone was staring at me. I became pretty paranoid. I wanted to walk around with a T-shirt saying: 'Yes, I do have cancer'; but I decided against it. I wore a wig but unfortunately it was obvious it was a wig and not my natural hair. I refused to wear bandanas; I just felt they didn't make me feel or look like a woman. Eventually, I came to terms with it and walked around without thinking about it. I didn't care – I was alive and I knew my hair would grow back one day. I even allowed my husband to take some photos of me without a wig. These are now photos I treasure and am so pleased with the results. My husband said I looked sexy, but I think he's just being kind.

I coped well with the treatment in general and was only sick once. One of the most embarrassing times was when I had a volunteer caring for me. We were talking and, just as I was about to say something, vomit not words came out of my mouth instead.

I felt so sorry for this poor young guy, but he acted as if it was a normal everyday thing. What a wonderful chap he was.

I had my stem cells harvested and put away for use later. Thankfully, I've never needed them.

It's now eight years since I've been free from cancer. I intend to be that way until I'm at least ninety. I have an annual check-up, an ultrasound, blood tests and CT scan. I get very emotional around this time, as the fear builds inside me, imagining lumps that aren't there. I think of all the times I haven't felt well since my last annual check-up and wonder if the cancer has returned. The moment the tests are over, I calm down and laugh at my craziness and go on living my life again.

I know mentally the experience of cancer will always be with me, for the rest of my life. But I have a great life and an interesting story to tell. Perhaps that's why I got the disease.

I like to share my story and listen to others and offer hope. I have a ribbon with the words 'Inspire Hope' tattooed on my tummy; this was my fifth anniversary gift to myself. It's a reminder I'm here and I'm well. Cancer is a word, not a sentence.

One day, hopefully, all this will be a very distant memory and I will be able to share it with my grandchildren with a smile. I will look back and remember I was chosen to have this disease and I came out the other side.

If I can do it, you can too.

CHRIS GEIGER

GUINNESS WORLD RECORD NEWSPAPER FEATURE

(FIRST PUBLISHED ON WORLD CANCER DAY)

Below is my special 'World Record' newspaper feature. Daily newspapers around the world supported me in publishing this feature. This enabled me to achieve a Guinness World Record and more importantly created much-needed cancer awareness around the world.

Congratulations! You're one of millions of people, in potentially 38 countries, reading this column today. You've also enabled me to make history, by becoming the first person to obtain a Guinness World Record for the *'most published feature newspaper article in one day – by the same author'*. You're reading this in one of hopefully 400 newspapers that have kindly agreed to help.

I have a romantic notion that you're reading this while sitting on a tram in Melbourne, or the subway in Manhattan, or while eating breakfast in your hotel in, say, Dubai. Some of you will no doubt be reading this in bed after a busy day, and sadly some will be reading it from a hospital bed; hospitals like the Worthing Hospital, or University College Hospital, in London.

Sadly, another thing that connects the millions of people reading this today is cancer. This terrible disease isn't fussy who it affects. It doesn't care which newspaper you read or where you read it.

There are more than 200 types of cancer, with around 12.7 million new cases diagnosed worldwide each year. More than 1 in 3 of us will get some form of cancer during our lifetime.

More people worry about cancer than debt, crime or losing their job. Scientists believe stress is one of the biggest contributory causes of cancer – along with habits such as smoking, overeating and heavy drinking.

I'm one of the lucky ones; nineteen years ago, I was diagnosed with a cancer called Non-Hodgkin Lymphoma, and given just three months to live. I had a tumour the size of a dinner plate, buried in the middle of my chest.

I spent eight months feeling dreadfully unwell, so was actually pleased when doctors put a name to it. Naively I hadn't realized that Non-Hodgkin Lymphoma was a form of cancer. I'd wrongly assumed I had an unusual condition that would be sorted out with a few pills.

While I was lying in a hospital bed, a nurse handed me a leaflet offering advice about cancer treatment. I later asked my doctor if lymphoma was cancer; this is when I was told the brutal truth.

I started writing a memoir about my experience, and the reaction from people around me was one of surprise when they found out. They always responded with positive comments, but the expression on their faces said, '*Why are you bothering?*'

I had most of the physical symptoms the cancer leaflet described, but equally I had a mental battle to win, if I was to remain positive.

A nurse suggested I keep my thoughts to myself, to help protect my family and friends. So I began writing, a way to offload my anxiety and remain focused.

I'd no idea of the sort of hell I was about to go through. I endured two years of treatment, which included radiotherapy, chemotherapy and a bone marrow transplant.

Despite the side effects of the treatment and what the doctors had said, I never once thought this lump in my chest would kill me. Writing my diary helped me stay positive. I'm 44 years old now.

It's not a coincidence I chose today to write this feature, or obtain a Guinness World Record; it's 'World Cancer Day'. On the 4th February every year, people, businesses, governments and the media work together, to create global cancer awareness and explore methods to prevent, detect and treat it.

With the help and support of the *Bristol Evening Post*, I've made history by creating the most published feature newspaper article in one day. More importantly, by reading this, it may just save your life. Don't worry, you'll not need to put your hand in your pocket, nor have the embarrassment of collecting sponsorship money from friends. It involves just a few simple steps, literally.

A review by Cancer Research-funded researchers at Bristol University revealed that, by simply exercising for just 30 minutes a day, you could cut the risk of bowel cancer by up to 50 percent. Exercise also helps prevent breast, lung and endometrial cancer. Even in these hard financial times, going for a walk costs nothing. Breast, lung, bowel and prostate cancers account for over half of all new cancers each year. Just think how many lives exercise alone could save.

The European Prospective Investigation into Cancer and Nutrition (EPIC) study has found that eating plenty of fruit and vegetables could reduce the risk of mouth, oesophageal and lung cancers, as well as some types of stomach cancer. Again, think how many lives could be saved by just eating vegetables.

If everyone did as I suggest above, perhaps I could obtain another World Record for saving the most lives; I'm obviously joking but a nice thought.

Cancer is a leading cause of death around the world, according to the World Health Organization, which estimates that 84 million people will die of cancer between 2005 and 2015 without intervention.

The good news, however, is cancer survival rates have doubled in the last 40 years. More than half the people diagnosed with cancer now survive their disease for more than five years. In men, the highest five-year survival rate is for testicular cancer, with a massive 95 percent of men surviving. For women, the highest five-year survival rate, at 90 percent, is for malignant melanoma.

So I've proven that it's easy to achieve things if we work together. Very easily, you've helped me achieve a Guinness World Record, by simply reading this column. I've also shown you that exercising for just 30 minutes a day can reduce some cancers by up to 50 percent. Just think what 'we', collectively, as a group of people worldwide could accomplish, if we work together to destroy this terrible disease.

I'm currently writing a book, a collection of true inspirational stories from cancer survivors like myself, who have battled to overcome the effects of this awful disease. I want the book to motivate, encourage and give hope to cancer sufferers, their families and friends.

Therefore, if you have an inspirational story to share, for possible publication, please contact me via my website: www. ChrisGeiger.com

GETTING INVOLVED

It's true what they say about the simplest ideas being the best. Shortly after my Guinness World Record feature was published, I received the following email.

From:	Tim [removed]
Sent:	5 February 2011 21:27
To:	Chris Geiger <Email@ChrisGeiger.co.uk>
Subject:	RE: Book – Inspiring Stories.

Dear Chris,

I have just read your amazing World Cancer Day feature, and wanted to say how inspiring and moving I found it. I've never responded to a newspaper article before, nor written to a stranger.

I am unfortunately not yet a cancer survivor, but a sufferer. I have been diagnosed with cancer of the rectum. I'm due to have an operation soon to have a tumour removed. I sincerely hope one day, I too will be a survivor like you, and be able to submit my story.

I share your thinking that such a book full of survivors' stories will really make a difference to those who have cancer – sufferers like hearing about people who have beaten this disease. Hope and strength are two very important things a cancer patient needs to become a survivor; your book provides both.

The awareness you're creating by your newspaper columns and your book idea will give hope to thousands.

I pray that one day I'm in a position to send you my survivor's story, to motivate and help others. Until then, God bless and keep up the great work.

Thanks and speak to you soon.

Tim

As you can imagine, this email was one of hundreds I received from around the world. However, I found this message particularly emotional. It cemented my idea that such a book would not only help and inspire people, but would also give readers and patients hope that one day they could have their story published. My goal now is to make this the first of a biannual publication.

When I was receiving treatment for cancer, I set myself goals, which gave me something to focus on. My hope is this book will also provide anyone affected by cancer something to focus their attention on. In addition, by patients sharing their stories, it helps those who read them.

Even if you think your writing won't win an award for its descriptive prose, don't worry – I'm happy to work with you to 'polish' your story.

If you or any member of your family has been touched

by cancer, I'd love to hear from you. Any story relating to cancer from anyone's perspective can be submitted. However, all stories must be true and make a positive impact.

I highly recommend you read your story out loud, as this helps bring out any errors and enables you to check the story flows. Anyone who tries to advertise or promote a product or service will not be included. Finally, I cannot, sadly, accept any story that is longer than 4,000 words.

You may submit your stories by email only. Each submission must include the following: your full name, postal address and phone number, together with your email address and title of the story.

In the subject line, enter 'Story Submission'. Copy and paste (or type) the story into the body of the email; no attachments will be accepted. One submission per email to: stories@ChrisGeiger.co.uk

Please direct any questions and suggestions to: info@ChrisGeiger.co.uk

CANCER-RELATED
WEBSITES & BLOGS

http://www.aicr.org.uk
Worldwide Cancer Research is a cancer charity that funds
research into cancer worldwide.

http://www.AboveAndBeyond.org.uk
A Bristol-based charity supporting local NHS hospitals.

http://www.AnthonyNolan.org
Information on stem cell transplants and becoming a bone
marrow donor.

http://www.BeatBloodCancers.org
Useful information on all types of lymphoma and
leukaemia.

http://www.BowelCancerUK.org.uk
Offers support and help for bowel cancer patients.

http://www.thebraintumourcharity.org
Advice for sufferers of brain tumours.

http://www.BreastCancerCare.org.uk
Support and help for those affected by breast cancer.

http://www.Cancer.gov
A comprehensive American cancer resource from the government's principal agency on cancer research.

http://www.CancerAdvice.co.uk
Details on various different types of cancer.

http://www.CancerInCommon.com
A social network where patients and survivors can connect based on their cancer type and location.

http://www.CancerResearchUK.org
Easy-to-understand cancer patient information.

http://www.TheCancerSurvivorsClub.com
The Cancer Survivors Club book website.

http://CaveCrawlerStory.blogspot.co.uk
Dave Mason's blog about his Pseudomyxoma Peritonei (PMP).

http://www.CheckEmLads.com
A testicular cancer awareness website.

http://www.ChrisGeiger.co.uk
Chris Geiger's official website.

http://www.HealthTalkOnline.org
A place to share any cancer experiences and concerns.

http://www.JosTrust.org.uk
Easy-to-understand information about cervical cancer.

http://www.LeukaemiaCare.org.uk
Blood cancer care and support.

http://www.LifePowerBlog.ca
Andrea Paine's blog inspires runners and cancer survivors alike.

http://www.Lymphomas.org.uk
Offers useful information on lymphoma and a chat room.

http://www.Macmillan.org.uk
Practical advice on living with cancer.

http://www.NHS.uk/conditions/cancer
Offers a guide to cancer treatment centres.

http://www.Orchid-Cancer.org.uk
Information on testicular, prostate and penile cancers.

http://www.PancreaticCancerAction.org
Information on pancreatic cancer
and the charity established by Ali Stunt.

http://www.PennyBrohnCancerCare.org
Offers free complementary therapies, advice and
counselling for those dealing with cancer.

http://www.PseudomyxomaSurvivor.co.uk
A support network for survivors and carers of
Pseudomyxoma Peritonei.

http://www.TeenageCancerTrust.org
A charity devoted to improving the lives of teenagers and
young adults with cancer.

http://www.Twitter.com/Cancer_Buzz
Providing daily news and information on anything cancer
related.

http://en.wikipedia.org/wiki/Cancer
A free encyclopedia, detailing the history and methods
used to treat cancer.

To add your website or blog to future editions, please submit
it to: URL@ChrisGeiger.co.uk

SURVIVORS UPDATE

Claire Duffett – In Sickness and in Health

Claire Duffett now lives back in Bristol with Richard, her husband. They enjoy family days out with their children, Ruby and Lola. Their interests include swimming, walking and reading. Ruby is doing well at her first school and Lola is looking forward to starting school soon. Witnessing her children attend school is a day Claire didn't think she would see, so has extra meaning. Claire remains cancer free some five years after treatment.

Ali Stunt – I'm a Statistic of One

Ali Stunt is entering her sixth year of survival after being diagnosed with pancreatic cancer. She considers herself incredibly lucky as only three percent of patients ever get this far. She is now devoting her time to running the charity she set up, called Pancreatic Cancer Action. The aim of this charity is to raise awareness and educate people about the disease. Her dream is that more people like her can have the same outcome. Ali enjoys spending time with her family, walking her two golden retrievers and having lots of laughs with her girlfriends! To date, recent scans and blood tests are still showing 'no evidence of disease'.

Katie Patterson – The Cancer Card

Katie Patterson went on to finish her studies at university and really enjoyed 'uni life'. She has a part-time job in a cocktail bar, which has brought her a whole new group of friends to have even more fun with. On finishing her treatment she enjoyed a girly holiday in Ibiza with her friends. Katie's second fund-raising fancy-dress walk was also a great success.

Katie recently celebrated being in remission for five years since her transplant. To mark this huge milestone she is currently backpacking around Australia.

Jason Edgar – My Journey

Jason Edgar lives with his daughter Holly. He works as part of a project team for a large health insurer. In his spare time, Jason is a cancer awareness campaigner and fundraiser for both local and national testicular cancer charities.

Jason enjoys time with his daughter and has recently got engaged to his new partner Sarah. His hobbies include swimming, walking and music festivals. Most importantly to him, he is part of his daughter's life. Jason is still cancer free and loves every moment of being a member of the cancer survivors club.

Kate Beynon – Animal Therapy

Kate Beynon continues to live in a beautiful part of Wales, on a dairy farm with her husband and energetic sons, Tom, Jack and Harry. She works on their farm and manages a small campsite, which keeps both her mind and body active. Living on the Gower for Kate is idyllic, especially being so close to the sea. She has an assortment of animals – cats, dogs, horses, cows and calves who are her therapy and counsellors. Kate also works hard in raising awareness and money for cancer charities. There are lasting complications from her treatment, which she deals with on a day-to-day basis; however, each morning when she wakes, she's grateful and always makes the most of it.

Jessica Smith – Life and Death Inside Me

Jessica Smith continues first and foremost to be a full-time mum to her two beautiful boys. She is the healthiest and fittest she has ever been and enjoys life tremendously.

Jessica and her family go camping whenever they can and she's making plans to start her own business once her younger son starts school. Jessica runs a playgroup, is part of her son's Parents Teacher Association and is totally immersed in family life. Jessica still has regular check-ups to monitor her side effects and her body after cancer but, six years on, she is delighted to say that her illness has not returned.

Marilyn Taylor – A Bright Light

Marilyn Taylor lives with her husband in Derbyshire and still enjoys the gardening that she credits with saving her life. She recently attended the marriage of her only daughter and likes to spend time with her grandson. Her newfound hobby is seeking out priceless treasures at car boot sales on Sunday mornings.

Michael Stephenson – A Father's Perspective

Michael's daughter Clare reached her seven-year milestone in August 2012. She is fit and well; the dark days are now a distant memory. This experience has really changed all their lives. Both Clare and Kris work hard to raise awareness for various local cancer charities near their home in Bristol. When not working together, running a printing business, their other hobbies include extending their house. No longer do Michael and Yvonne take life for granted; they appreciate just how precious life is.

Andrea Paine – Things Happen for a Reason

Andrea Paine is a Senior Director for the Federal Minister of Health in Ottawa, Canada. She lives in Montreal, Quebec, with her husband and three daughters. An avid runner, she is always training for various races and half-marathons.

Her blog is continuing to inspire both cancer survivors and runners alike. Andrea remains cancer free and has a more positive outlook on life than ever.

Paula Glass – Live Life to the Full

Paula Glass is now at work full-time after having to start gradually. She has recently purchased her first home and still enjoys socializing and having day trips out with friends. After completing her cancer treatment, she is feeling better than she ever has before and is still cancer free.

Julie King – If in Doubt, Persevere

Julie King lives in Cheshire with her husband and two teenage sons. She has decided not to return to teaching and thoroughly enjoys her voluntary work. Her hobbies include gardening, reading, swimming and yoga. She is currently busy project managing the renovation of a house she and her husband recently bought. Since her treatment finished, she remains well and cancer free. She is delighted to report that people tell her she looks better than she did in her pre-cancer days, which she attributes to a different outlook on life and continuation of the healthier diet she adopted during treatment.

Mark Davies – How to Solve a Problem like my Rear

It has been seven years since Mark successfully underwent Papillon radiotherapy and TEM micro-surgery, and he is still free of cancer. Having closed his company after diagnosis, Mark now works part-time for the company that makes the Papillon machine as its patient advocate, as well as giving lectures to bowel cancer screening nurses at various conferences. He has written his own cancer story and shares his experiences as a patient voice with patients, carers and survivors. He went travelling for six months after the five-year all clear to South-East Asia, Australia and New Zealand, and now lives in Manchester.

Amanda Baird – Never Give Up

Amanda had another disease-free MRI scan last June and just has a check-up every six months. She successfully completed the triathlon she mentioned in a time of one hour seventeen minutes, which was a huge personal achievement for her and helped raised a lot of money for Pancreatic Cancer UK. Her cycle ride from London to Brighton will go ahead in September of this year. She is feeling fabulous and looking to the future with optimism and hope.

Helen Gorick – Miracles Do Happen

Helen Gorick lives in Devon with her husband, Mark, and children from her first marriage. She is running her own business making glass beads and also teaches others. When not in her studio, she enjoys walking her dogs on the beautiful Devon coastline. Her other hobbies include nature photography. Nearly eight years after her stem cell transplant, she remains cancer free.

Abbie Sparks – Better You than Me

Abbie Sparks lives in Bristol with her mum and is training to become a paramedic. She enjoys horse riding, going to the gym and generally being alive. More than fourteen years after her treatment, she is still cancer free and remains very positive.

David Mason – Mother of All Surgeries

David Mason lives with his wife, Tracey, and two daughters, Jessica and Chloe. David has made a return to caving, climbing, fishing and running, and ran a half-marathon, raising funds for research into Pseudomyxoma Peritonei. He is also looking forward to his first family holiday since his treatment.

Gillian Metcalfe – A Mother's Perspective

If it hadn't been for Alessandro getting sick, his natural talent for playing the piano would never have been discovered. He still wakes up every morning and plays even before his breakfast. He's won a few awards including the award for best young musician of the year in Gibraltar and has formed a band with his friends. He has played in quite a few local clubs and his ambition now is to do well in his A-levels and go to a music university to further his knowledge. It's been seven years since his treatment and he is now a very healthy young man.

Barbara Conway – How It Was

Barbara has now been discharged from hospital; she celebrated in style with a glass of wine. Currently, she is working four days a week as an Accounts Manager for a small family business. She also teaches children to dance and is a qualified colour counsellor and healer, teacher and colour life coach. Barbara enjoys having holidays by the sea and visiting her brother and his wife in the Lake District. She also loves going out with friends and family and spending time with her two cats who helped her when she was having treatment for cancer.

Mark Gillett – Keep Smiling

Mark Gillett is married with two children: Sam, a lovely boy aged ten, and Sophie, a six-year-old bundle of energy. He works in a local college, which is challenging but fun, and, while still living with diabetes, he will never forget the past, and he is very positive about the future and looking forward to the coming years.

Kathleen Giles – Too Frightened to Ask

Kathleen has just celebrated her silver wedding anniversary and loves spending time with her two rapidly growing grand-children. She has been cancer free since 1995.

Stewart Hodge – Getting the Gist

It's now nearly five years since Stewart finished his treatment. He still feels extremely fortunate that a young doctor, whom he never met again, correctly sensed he had a tumour. He feels in a privileged position to have beaten the disease, something he'll never take for granted again. The simplest things, like spending time with his family, give him the most pleasure.

Shelly Ostrouhoff – Cancer Is a Word, Not a Sentence

A recent scan confirmed that Shelly Ostrouhoff has now been free of cancer for over ten years. She looks forward to spending the rest of her long life with her two children and husband, Michael, on the Gold Coast in Australia, enjoying the simple things in life. Sadly, her sister was recently diagnosed with breast cancer, so she is now using her knowledge and experience to help her overcome the disease – we look forward to reading her survival story in the next edition!